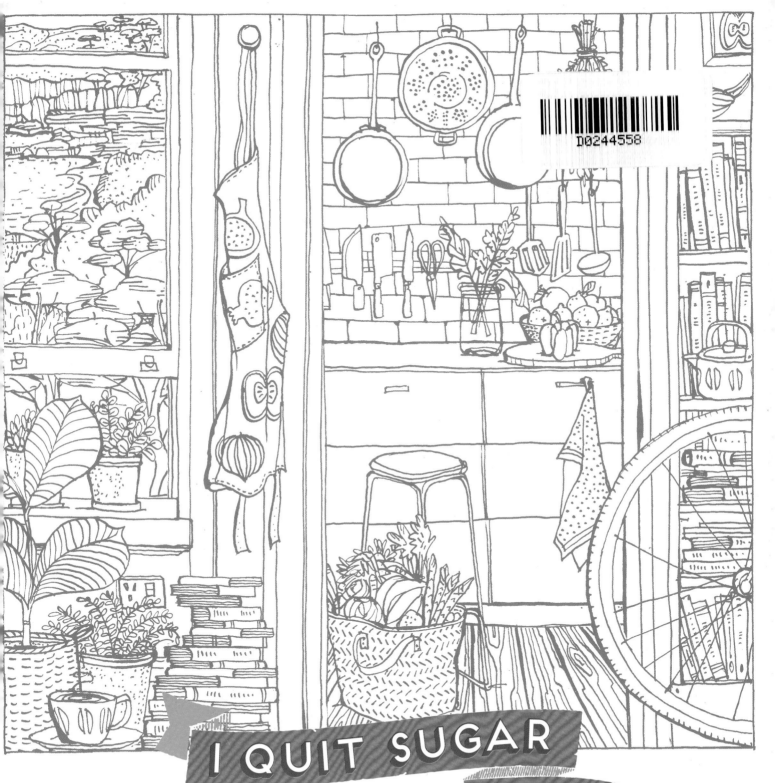

I QUIT SUGAR

FOR LIFE

This is my follow-up book to help
make cooking, eating and our health
more elegant and joyous.

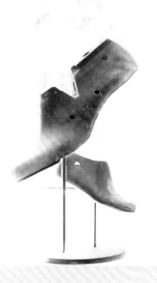

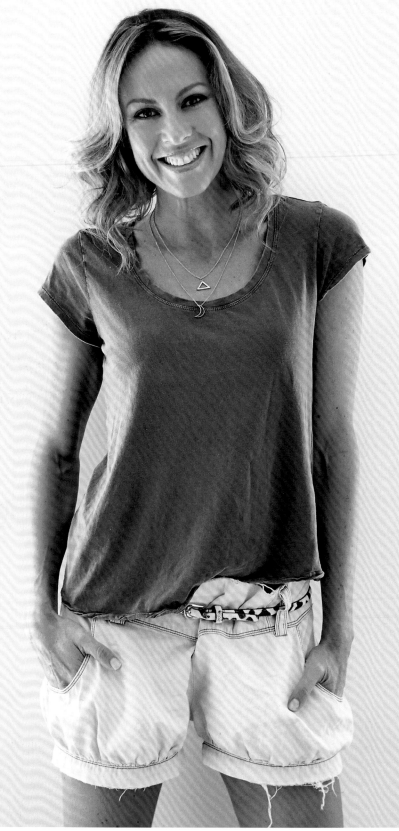

I QUIT SUGAR

FOR LIFE

Your FAD-FREE
WHOLEFOOD WELLNESS CODE
and COOKBOOK

SARAH WILSON

MACMILLAN

First published 2014 by
Macmillan Australia

This edition first published in the UK 2014
by Pan Macmillan UK, an imprint of Pan Macmillan,
a division of Macmillan Publishers Limited
Pan Macmillan, 20 New Wharf Road, London N1 9RR
Basingstoke and Oxford
Associated companies throughout the world
www.panmacmillan.com

ISBN 978-1-4472-7334-9

Photography © Marija Ivkovic 2014
Illustrations © Kat Chadwick 2014
Photography by Marija Ivkovic
Additional photography courtesy of Sarah Wilson
Styling by Lee Blaylock
Additional styling by Sarah Wilson
Food preparation by Lee Blaylock and Rochelle Seator
Design and typesetting by Trisha Garner
Additional design by Debra Billson
Additional typesetting by Post Pre-press Group and James Garner
Editing by Samantha Sainsbury and Nicola Young
Additional recipes by Martyna Angell
Illustrations by Kat Chadwick
Index by Puddingburn Publishing Services

1 3 5 7 9 8 6 4 2

A CIP catalogue record for this book is available from the British Library.

Printed in Italy by Rotolito Lombarda SpA

Visit **www.panmacmillan.com** to read more about all our books and to buy them.
You will also find features, author interviews and news of any author events,
and you can sign up for e-newsletters so that you're always first to hear
about our new releases.

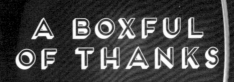

A BOXFUL OF THANKS

To the **250,000** (and counting) **SUGAR QUITTERS** who have given this experiment a crack.

THANKS.

You made me keep on keeping on. Mostly on my toes! Thank you for your questions and for challenging me robustly and often. You delivered me my dharma, which is the greatest gift a girl can be given.

Also, a BPA-free bucketful of gratitude to:

Jo Foster and photographer Marija Ivkovic for exceeding their briefs (sorry, Dad gag!) and caring. Always caring. Plus, Zoe and the I Quit Sugar team for boarding the train with swags of enthusiasm.

Also to the Pan Macmillan team – publisher Ingrid Ohlsson (for sticking by me and being a kindred spirit), editor Sam Sainsbury, big boss Cate Paterson and publicity whizz Charlotte Ree. Kat Chadwick for her fun illustrations. And Trisha and Deb for making things so pretty under pretty tight deadlines.

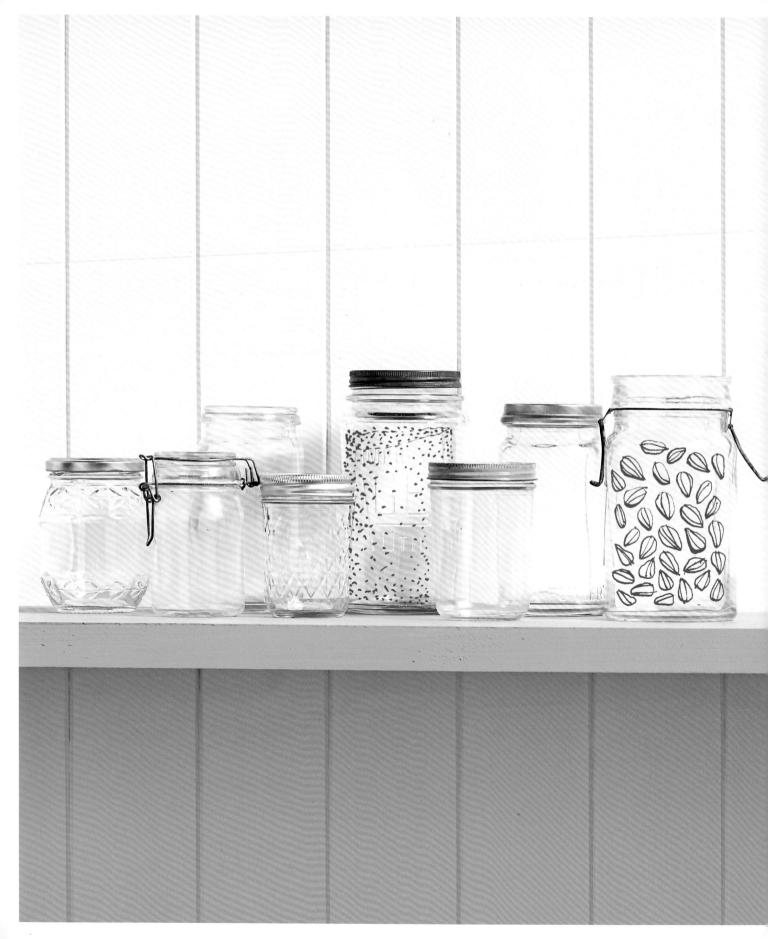

CONTENTS

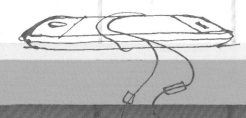

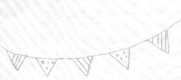

AN INVITATION

Dearest Reader,
You are cordially invited to join me
for a sugar-free life experiment.
It's a casual, all-day affair with a gentle vibe.
No fanfare, no fancy rules, open-toed shoes acceptable.

When I first quit sugar, I treated it as an invitation to try out a new way of living, just to – you know – see how it went. It went well, thanks! My health was transformed and in a matter of weeks I experienced a mood change. Actually, more accurately, I experienced a mood stabilisation. Since quitting sugar I've experienced a steady, calm happiness that has previously eluded me. I then shared how I did it with an eight-week detox programme, and a stack of you joined me at the party. Three years on and I'm asked almost hourly, 'So you quit . . . *then* what happened?'

The expectation, I think, is that surely by now I'd have toppled off the wagon and descended into a guilty, sugary pit. Because that's the value we give to diets, right? They work for a bit, but then self-control packs it in and we tumble back to base, having nasty chats in our head on the way down.

But this is the thing I've learned from my new, gentler way of living:

QUITTING SUGAR IS NOT A DIET.

It's not about crazy draconian rules and restrictive one-off weight-loss stunts. Indeed, it can be distilled into two supremely sensible concepts I reckon we all just *get*, intuitively:

 ## QUITTING SUGAR IS A WAY OF LIVING WITHOUT PROCESSED FOOD.

When you steer yourself away from sugar, it – by necessity – cuts out pretty much everything that comes in a packet or box. When people baulk at my no-sugar status, I calmly point out that I simply don't eat crap. It's that elegant.

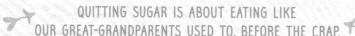 ## QUITTING SUGAR IS ABOUT EATING LIKE OUR GREAT-GRANDPARENTS USED TO. BEFORE THE CRAP.

This – again by necessity – sees us eating whole, un-mucked-with foods that were commonplace before the advent of modern metabolic diseases. One hundred years ago we ate 1 kg sugar a year, now we eat 60 kg a year. One hundred years ago we ate eggs for breakfast, meat at lunch, vegetables prepared simply, fruit as a treat and drank our milk whole. One hundred years ago type 2 diabetes, obesity, heart disease and cholesterol issues were rare if not non-existent.

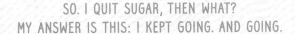

SO. I QUIT SUGAR, THEN WHAT?
MY ANSWER IS THIS: I KEPT GOING. AND GOING.

It's kind of like the way I treat going for a jog. If I pledge myself to a hard-core 1-hour run, I baulk. But if I gently commit to a 20-minute shuffle around the park in the sun, I do it . . . and chances are, because it feels pretty good, I keep going. And going. And, effortlessly, it becomes a 40-minute 'workout'.

Over time, I've let these principles that guide my eating – of experimenting, crowding out crap with better options and being gentle – unfurl a little further. And they began to inform the way I exercise, shop, make decisions (from what dental floss to buy to what city I'll live in next) and the way I keep my life balanced and meaningful.

As my oldest mate, Ragni, said,

'WHEN YOU QUIT SUGAR THERE'S NO TURNING BACK.
YOU CAN'T UNLEARN THIS STUFF. I MEAN, YOU NEVER FORGET THAT
A GLASS OF APPLE JUICE CONTAINS 10 TEASPOONS OF SUGAR.'

AND YOU CAN'T STOP IT FROM TAKING YOU FURTHER.
I Quit Sugar for Life is for everyone who wants to keep going. And going. It's for everyone who wants life to be simple, gentle and . . . *whole*. Honestly, I've written this book for my friends with kids (begging for no-fuss food and health tricks to get their family on a good track) and for all my solo mates who want to be well without the gimmicky diet palaver. Also, for everyone wanting to tread more sustainably on the planet, for this is the guts of *real* and whole wellness. My friend Georgia said to me recently, 'Just tell me what the hell we're meant to eat and do now . . . not what we *can't* eat and do.'

'OK,' I said. 'I'll write another book.'

I'm not a scientist. I'm a human guinea pig. And an impatient, busy one, hell-bent on finding the smoothest slipstream through life. I don't like fuss or bother or strictures. I'm not setting down rules. Nope, I'm issuing you an invitation to steer your choices away from sugar. And crap.

With this book, my experimenting has led to a 'Wellness Code' that I'll be outlining shortly. You can choose to follow it closely, or simply use it as a pivot point for reflecting on how to live well your *own* way. Always, always, I wish all of us to go our *own* way, listening to our *own* bodies, responding to our *own* needs.

- ✂

Note: This invitation is totally transferable. There's no expiry date.
RSVP: To yourself, if you're keen to keep going.

Lifelong, simple and whole wellness
to you all,

Sarah xx

PS: If you're yet to quit sugar, you might find *I Quit Sugar: Your Complete 8-Week Detox Program and Cookbook* helpful. Or you can do the online 8-Week Program at www.iquitsugar.com

I QUIT SUGAR FOR LIFE

. . . and this is how I've been going

Please don't think of me as a beacon of self-discipline. I'm not. Other people who've done my programme seem to be far more that way. They tell me they haven't touched a speck of the white stuff in six months. I'm in awe!

But then, I don't go for restriction. I prefer to let my body choose what it wants, confident that now that it's not addicted to sugar, it will naturally choose what's best.

THIS IS THE ULTIMATE AIM OF QUITTING SUGAR: TO RETURN TO OUR NATURAL APPETITE, LIKE WHEN WE WERE YOUNG KIDS.

AND WHEN YOU ACHIEVE IT . . . GOLLY, IT'S FOOD FREEDOM!

A study published through the American Psychological Association found self-control is a limited resource we need to manage through our day so that it doesn't get worn out too early. The scientists advise limiting the number of restrictive mandates in our lives to save our self-control muscle for the stuff that really matters. So: don't diet. Save your muscle for matters of love, career and travel, and who you want to be in life.

> Quitting sugar has given me a freedom from food that I never could have imagined. I finally realised it's not about willpower, it's a real addiction.   SAMANTHA

This is how it's worked out for me:
YEP, I 'LAPSE'. I ate a piece of homemade chocolate birthday cake recently. It *tasted* great. Then it *felt* overwhelmingly wrong. My ears and eyes and toenails buzzed. I felt *scratchy* and nauseous. Some might call this lapsing. I call it checking in. I cover this off soon in the Wellness Code (see page 7).

I TRAVEL SUGAR-FREE. For the bulk of my time off sugar I've been traipsing around the world, investigating better ways to eat whole and well, and writing more books along the way. I can now navigate airline food, Parisian breakfast buffets and New York delis with ease.

> I quit sugar in May this year and so far have lost 29 kg [over 4 stone] and counting!   VANESSA

I STILL BINGE. Occasionally. And get food-moody. No point my being too Pollyanna. I have a tumultuous history of emotional eating and overeating in general and have struggled for years to sit comfortably with my body. Thing is, I now turn to savoury comfort foods. Which means, mercifully, the 'binges' are very short-lived – fats and proteins (nut butter straight from the jar is my thing) fill you up before things get really out of control.

I EAT FRUIT. Yep, one to two pieces of *whole* fruit a day, mostly low-fructose berries and kiwifruit. I encourage cutting fruit out on the 8-week programme – it contains 1–4 teaspoons of sugar apiece – so that your body can recalibrate. I then encourage reintroducing whole fruit and seeing how you react. To be honest, low-fructose fruit like kiwifruit, berries or grapefruit is the best option.

FRUIT IS GREAT AS A TREAT. AND ONLY EVER WHOLE (NOT DRIED OR JUICED).

Bear in mind: fruit contains more fructose than it did a few generations back (it's being bred to be sweeter), and the idea of eating 4 pieces of fruit a day is a new notion. My grandmother ate fruit as a sweet treat. I do too now, opting to get my fibre and vitamins from vegetables.

I EAT SUGAR DAILY. WAIT? *What?* Yep, I eat fruit, and I'll have a few squares of 70% cocoa chocolate from time to time, even some honey. I guess it comes to about 5–8 teaspoons a day, sometimes more. I don't tally, but let my natural appetite tell me how much feels right. And this is the point: I'm conscious of what I'm eating and maintain a balance.

I CHOOSE HOW I TAKE MY SUGAR; I'M NOT FORCE-FED IT.

I know when it's too much. And I back off before the addiction kicks in. I'm armed with the info now . . . 'and you can't unlearn this stuff'. You just keep on using it to steer your choices.

I DON'T SHOP AT THE SUPERMARKET. Well, only about once a fortnight for loo paper and a few tins of tuna. I just don't eat stuff from packets or boxes. You don't when you quit sugar.

I EAT EXACTLY WHAT I WANT. No deprivation, ever. I eat abundantly and freeeeeely!

I EAT THREE MEALS A DAY. Very little snacking. More on this to come . . .

I'M NO LONGER SICK. As I've shared a few times, my Hashimoto's thyroiditis (an auto-immune disease affecting the thyroid gland) is what saw me quit sugar in the first place. It pretty much crippled me a few years ago, some side effects of which included: whacked-out blood sugar, screwed-up hormones, a predisposition to diabetes and high cholesterol, mood fluctuations, weakness to the point of not being able to work or walk for nine months, weight gain and much more. All of the above are now stable or overcome. I will have to manage my disease for the rest of my life. But I can do this now and live a long, well life, something others with my disease, including my uncle and grandmother, were not able to do. I've wiped out my antibody markers, something my doctors find astounding. Quitting sugar did this. It also instilled me with a calm, stable head and happiness.

I DOUBT MYSELF OFTEN. Which is a good thing; it keeps me experimenting and learning and alive to the issue.

> @ I have reversed my pre-diabetic state and reduced my thyroxine dosage from 300 micrograms daily to 50 micrograms or less a day. JACKIE

THREE MORE MANTRAS

When I first quit sugar, I worked to four mantras that kept me focused on why I was doing this crazy thing:

IQS MANTRA 1.

BE KIND AND GENTLE.
We live with care; we don't 'punish' ourselves into doing things.

IQS MANTRA 2.

REPLACE SUGAR WITH FAT.
To satiate, fuel and provide us with fun foods to eat.

IQS MANTRA 3.

FIND YOUR BLANK SLATE.
This is the whole point – to get our bodies back to their natural appetite so that we live according to what they need, not crave.

IQS MANTRA 4.

CROWDING OUT.
Eat so much of the good stuff that there's no room for the bad stuff (because we humans are better at doing rather than restricting!).

Now, down the track, I've added a few more:

▶ EAT DENSE (SEE PAGE 28)

▶ BACK THE FORK OFF (SEE PAGE 36)

▶ FLOW (SEE PAGE 46)
Yep, it's all about getting us some flow!

> I feel lighter and no longer bloated. Most importantly, I'm not sneaking around shoving sugar into my mouth any chance I get. MELANIE

The deal with SUGAR and AGEING

I RECENTLY TRAVELLED TO TWO OF THE WORLD'S FIVE BLUE ZONES (REGIONS WHERE PEOPLE LIVE THE LONGEST) – IKARIA IN GREECE AND SARDINIA IN ITALY. I joined a National Geographic team in Ikaria to look at what foods might be responsible for their robust, healthy and very long lives. What did we find? The locals eat an abundance of whole fats, proteins and seasonal vegetables. Oh, and they eat very little sugar.

According to the latest science, sugar reacts with proteins in our bodies, changing their structure to form toxic advanced glycation end-products (AGEs), which accelerate the ageing process. Sugar makes collagen and elastin less supple, radiant, elastic and resilient, and more susceptible to sun damage – just to complete the saggy picture. *Me, my skin changed dramatically when I quit, within weeks.* I have fewer wrinkles now than I did five years ago. Many other quitters report the same.

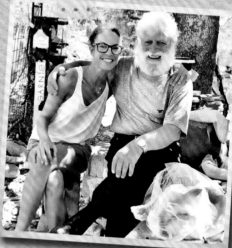

This Ikarian farmer is in his 90s, drinks ½ litre of wine at lunch and has a handshake of a sumo wrestler!

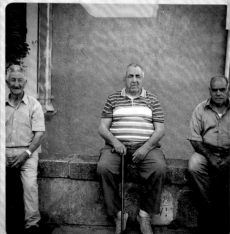

A sense of belonging and keeping good company are also Blue Zone longevity factors.

These Sardinian old timers show how it's done in a town in Nuoro where there are more centenarians than anywhere else on the planet.

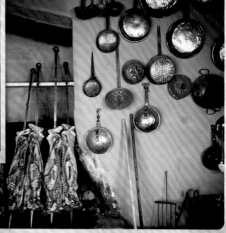

THE OTHER FACTORS I NOTED:
- Daily rest, daily red wine (with meals),
- Walking as transport,
- Seasonal food and not rushing.

All lifestyle approaches I wholeheartedly subscribe to in this book.

According to Dan Buettner, author of *The Blue Zones*, there's one distinguishing food all the Zones have in common – PORK. In Sardinia they slow roast it. In Ikaria they drink pork broth for vitality. Okinawans – lauded as the longest lived of all – are the only Japanese people to eat pork regularly. One Japanese scientist speculates it's because pigs are genetically similar to humans and that something in pork protein helps repair arterial damage.

I QUIT SUGAR FOR LIFE

I feel it's important to familiarise ourselves with the 'scientific' battle currently playing out in journals and blog forums around the globe as it's one we're going to be drawn into a lot more in coming years. This battle is predicted to get bloodier than the one we had with Big Tobacco a generation back. I'm hoping it's shorter.

On one side of the ring we have Big Food. Big Food likes us to eat sugar; it keeps their products cheap and highly addictive. Our health is not their priority, funnily enough! Big Food is very much in the corner. They've ridden off cheap sugar subsidies and the popularity of the low-fat movement (which necessitates adding sugar to make up for loss of flavour and texture) for decades and they don't want to back down. Their tactics are awe-inspiring. Their nimblest, so far: funding national nutrition bodies and paying individual dietitians to endorse sugar in the public domain. (And, in some cases, to publicly refute the work of people like me. Sigh.)

▶ In New York, a ban on super-sized sodas was met with a multimillion-dollar campaign by the soft-drink industry. The ban was reversed by the courts.

▶ Indeed, in the United States, 24 states, five cities and the US Congress have all floated initiatives in the past four years to tax sugary beverages. All have failed due to industry pressure.

▶ The Academy of Nutrition and Dietetics (which calls itself the world's largest organisation of food and nutrition professionals) is sponsored by Coca-Cola, Kellogg's and PepsiCo.

▶ The American Society for Nutrition is sponsored by Coca-Cola, Kellogg's, McDonald's, Nestlé, PepsiCo and the Sugar Association Inc.

▶ The Dietitians Association of Australia (DAA) is sponsored by Arnott's, Kellogg's and Nestlé.

A picture forms, right? And yet . . .
We have a hulking – and growing – body of science proving that what we thought we knew about sugar (a natural part of life, at worst, a harmless bunch of empty calories?) is wrong. Sugar is toxic, and the proof is rolling in study by study.

▶ Findings from a recent study show that in countries where people have greater access to sugar there are higher levels of diabetes.

▶ Drinking just one can of soft drink a day increases your risk of diabetes by 22%.

▶ Yale University researchers have shown that sugar is making us eat more, while three animal studies show it's more addictive than cocaine.

▶ A Harvard School of Public Health study has linked sugar to heart disease.

▶ Sugar increases risk of cancer according to a systematic review by the University of Maryland. A UCLA study shows cancer cells use fructose for tumour growth.

▶ And countless studies show sugar is directly linked to obesity. Few authorities now dispute this, a recent development since I first began this IQS journey.

Are we eating less or more sugar?
More. Much more. But this is weird: in 2011, two Australian nutrition and diabetes experts published a study arguing that at the same time obesity rates soared (tripling in 30 years), consumption of refined sugar had fallen. They called this phenomenon 'the Australian Paradox' in an effort to show sugar is OK to eat. And, yes, I did just tell you they're diabetes experts.

The only issue is, there is no Australian Paradox. Indeed, the crux of the case rested on data that doesn't even exist. The Australian Bureau of Statistics aborted the survey more than a decade ago because it was unreliable, something they only do in cases where the data is so flimsy. In fact, a recently published study by the University of Western Australia over a 22-year period showed very large increases in the consumption of sugar in our nation. In fact, Australian Import data shows average sugar consumption from imported food alone is 30 g per day per person!

▶▶▷ LET'S TRY THIS ◁◀◀
TAKE CONTROL OF OUR WELLNESS

There's no point waiting around for laws to change or dietary guidelines to shift. As the National Health and Medical Research Council (NHMRC) chair said when announcing the changes to the Australian Dietary Guidelines: 'The challenge is there's so many people out there in the community that have got a vested interest.' We have to change ourselves. That's OK. In fact, it's more empowering this way. We can vote with our dollar and unlearn the vested information ourselves.

This ain't no flash-in-the-pan fad. Nope, it's a powerful way of life. Want some pointers on how it can be done? Flick on . . .

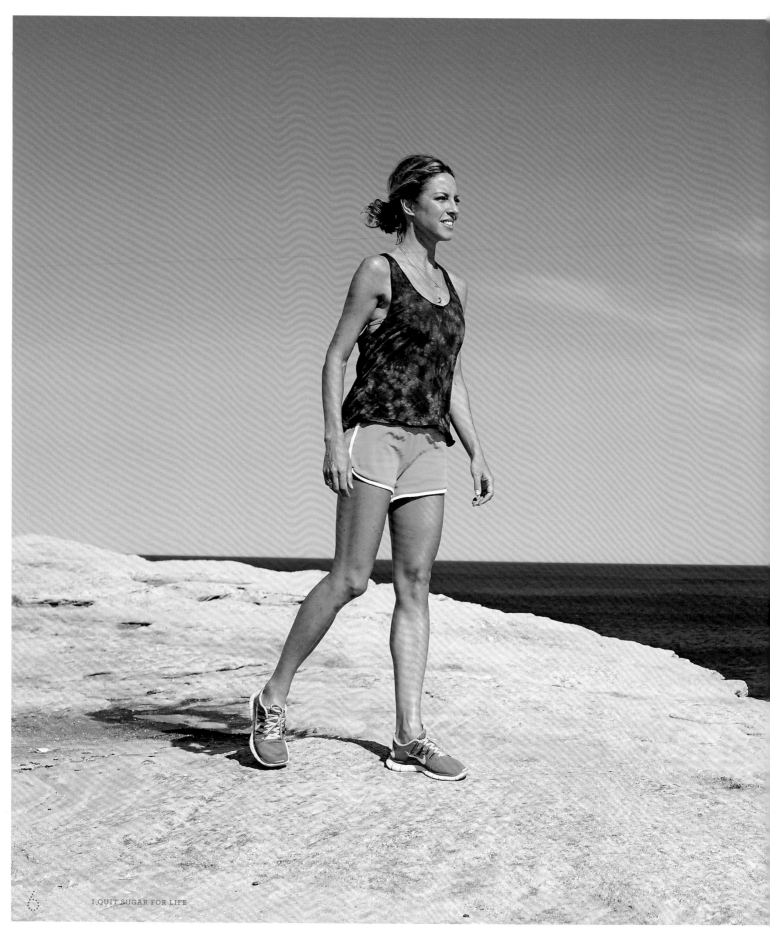

I QUIT SUGAR FOR LIFE

THE
I QUIT SUGAR
WELLNESS CODE

I see this 9-part code as a framework for simple, no-brainer health that supports sugar-free living.

It's assembled from interviews I've conducted with the world's leading wellness experts and from my health theories. Digest and then turn to the four-week programme to start your own wellness experiment.

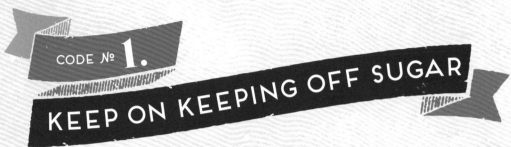

KEEP ON KEEPING OFF SUGAR

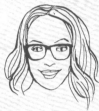

AFTER YOU'VE QUIT SUGAR WITH THE
EIGHT-WEEK PROGRAMME you pretty
much continue quitting sugar.

LET'S GO OVER THE GIST AGAIN:

Do we need sugar?

We need *glucose*, for sure. But not fructose. As paediatric endocrinologist Dr Robert Lustig says, 'There is not one biochemical reaction in your body, not one, that requires dietary fructose, not one that requires sugar. Dietary sugar is completely irrelevant to life. People say, oh, you need sugar to live. Garbage.' In addition: 58% of protein and 10% of fat changes into glucose once in the body, which can be used as needed. In fact, even if you *only* ate meats, eggs and good fats, you'd easily fulfil all of your body's glucose needs.

How much sugar are we meant to eat again?

As little as possible is the short answer. The longer answer is more convoluted and there are many diverging opinions on intake and what constitutes sugar and, indeed, added sugar.

Around the world, recommendations are increasingly being revised down and down, which suggests something, right? The American Heart Foundation's 2013 recommendations (revised down) advise no more than 5 teaspoons (20 grams) a day for women, 9 teaspoons (36 grams) for men and 3 teaspoons (12 grams) for kids.

The British Dietetic Association recommends about 50 grams or 12 teaspoons a day. The World Health Organisation (WHO) recently advised this figure should be lower following reviews of the scientific evidence of the link with obesity. However, the UK government's scientific advisory committee on nutrition – whose senior members advising on the sugar issue also work for large sugar companies – is fighting this (surprised much?).

The European Heart Network in 2011 set the aim of limiting intake to 6 teaspoons.

In Australia, there are no government recommendations on sugar intake, but the latest Australian Dietary Guidelines (2013) revised down their sugar intake message from 'eat moderately' to 'limit', again in response to the mounting scientific evidence against sugar.

Where does this leave us? As a general rule, I simply try to keep my sugar intake as low as possible. If pressed for a limit? I work to what many argue is the amount we ate back when our metabolisms were forming 10,000 years ago, derived from a few pieces of fruit and starches. It's an imprecise but useful target:

5–9 TEASPOONS OF ADDED SUGAR A DAY IS MY RECOMMENDED LIMIT.

How do we keep to this limit?

As part of IQS, we avoid foods that contain sugar.
Which sugars?
Any comprised of fructose:

- table sugar (sucrose) 50% fructose
- high-fructose corn syrup (HFCS) 55% fructose
- agave 70–90% fructose (I know, I know, the health food shops love this stuff, but it's a marketing con that's convinced everyone it's healthy and low-GI)
- honey 40% fructose
- maple syrup 35% fructose
- coconut and palm sugars 35–45% fructose.

We substitute with safe sweeteners.

The recipes in this book use the only two sweeteners my research has found to be safe and that are also easy to cook with:

STEVIA, which contains stevioside (300 times sweeter than sugar) and rebaudioside (450 times sweeter than sugar). It's a natural alternative, derived from the leaf of the stevia plant, and contains no fructose.

RICE MALT SYRUP (sometimes called rice syrup or brown rice syrup, particularly in the US), a natural sweetener that is made from fermented cooked rice and is a blend of complex carbohydrates, maltose and glucose. It's a relatively slow-releasing sweetener so it doesn't dump on the liver as much as pure glucose does. Make sure the ingredients list only rice (and water). Some versions add extra (fructose-containing) sugars.

OTHER SWEETENERS THAT ARE OK TO USE IN MODERATION are **xylitol** (a sugar alcohol that can be digested by our bodies) and **dextrose** (100% glucose).

I don't personally use pure glucose in my recipes, instead opting for the rice malt syrup which is a slower (and gentler) release. I find recipes that call for glucose/dextrose use a lot of it (cups instead of tablespoons!) – be careful of this.

THE REST: DON'T TOUCH. Most have been shown to be either carcinogenic or entirely indigestible, thus causing myriad health issues (um, ever noticed how 'sugar-free' gum can make you loose-bowelled and gassy?!). Many of the fake sugars available are banned in parts of Europe, deemed unsafe. Nuff said.

BEWARE

EVEN NON-FRUCTOSE SUGARS, SUCH AS GLUCOSE, ARE NOT GOOD TO EAT IN LARGE QUANTITIES AND WILL CAUSE INSULIN WOBBLINESS TOO, ALBEIT IN A FAR MORE MANAGEABLE WAY. WHAT'S MORE, STUDIES AT THE UNIVERSITY OF WASHINGTON HAVE FOUND THAT CONSUMING *ANY* KIND OF SWEETENER – EVEN THE 'FAKE' ONES THAT DON'T CONTAIN ANY KIND OF SUGAR – CAN CAUSE A BLOOD SUGAR SPIKE AND CONTINUE A SUGAR ADDICTION. JUST THE SWEET TASTE CAN TRIGGER INSULIN AND METABOLIC RESPONSES.

Q. WHAT'S THE DEAL WITH LOW-GI?

We hear a lot about low-GI foods. It's a ranking of carbohydrates that determines the extent to which blood sugar levels are raised after eating those foods. A 'low-GI' reading (readings under 55) is meant to be a good thing.

But want to know one of the 'best' ways a manufacturer can reduce their product's GI? *Add fructose.*

Fructose is one of the lowest GI substances around. Which is why Nutella has a lower GI than a carrot.

True story. For this reason I, and many health advisors, including Australia's NHMRC as of 2013, give little credence to low-GI as a nutritional guide.

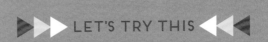

LET'S TRY THIS

MINIMISE ALL SWEETNESS

Granted, I like to play with fructose-free desserts and treats. However, going sugar-free for life means you'll need to:

EAT 'SWEET' TREATS AS TREATS ONLY. Even when a recipe contains a safe sweetener, it should be eaten with care. Not without other nutrients and fibre, not in large quantities and preferably not every day, unless they're sweetened with coconut oil, flesh, cream or milk only.

SLASH YOUR SWEETENER. I tend to use a very small amount of stevia or rice malt syrup in my recipes, but there's room for you to cut back even further.

You see, once you've quit sugar, your sweet point shifts. Try to shift it even lower.

SUGAR STACKS:
As part of IQS, we are super-careful with the hidden sugars.

Because the obvious sugar (a cube in your coffee) ain't nothing compared to these seductive doozies:

► **BARBECUE SAUCE = 4 TEASPOONS OF SUGAR IN A SERVE OF SAUCE ON YOUR MEAL**

FACT: Packaged sauces are often 50% sugar.

► **MUESLI BAR = 3–5 TEASPOONS OF SUGAR PER BAR**

FACT: Even the ones that are labelled 'sugar free'. The dried fruit deems them a fructose bomb!

► **A LOW-FAT YOGHURT (SINGLE SERVE) = 6½ TEASPOONS OF SUGAR**

FACT: When manufacturers take the fat out, they put sugar in to make up for lost flavour and texture, often disguised with other names, such as inulin and oligofructose.

► **A SMALL PACKET OF SULTANAS = 8 TEASPOONS OF SUGAR**

FACT: Bars with dried fruit contain up to 70% sugar.

► **APPLE JUICE = 10 TEASPOONS OF SUGAR PER GLASS**

FACT: A glass of apple juice contains the same amount of sugar as a glass of Coke.

► **TOMATO PASTA SAUCE = 10–12 TEASPOONS OF SUGAR PER SERVE**

FACT: 'Savoury' dinner sauces often contain more sugar than chocolate topping, particularly the tomato-based ones.

REMEMBER

IF YOU'RE IN THE PROCESS OF QUITTING SUGAR ON MY 8-WEEK PROGRAMME . . .

I ADVISE NO SWEETNESS AT ALL – INCLUDING STEVIA AND RICE MALT SYRUP AND LOW-FRUCTOSE FRUIT (COCONUT PRODUCTS ARE OK) – UNTIL WEEK SIX OF THE EIGHT-WEEK PROGRAMME. THIS IS TO RECALIBRATE YOUR BODY AND ARREST THE SWEET ADDICTION.

SAME IF YOU'RE 'RECALIBRATING' AFTER A BIT OF A LAPSE. GO COMPLETELY SAVOURY FOR A FEW DAYS, TO REST YOUR PALATE AND TO GET OFF THE SWEET CRAVINGS CYCLE. SELECT RECIPES AND FOODS ACCORDINGLY. AT THE END OF THIS PROCESS, I LIKE TO SLOWLY REINTRODUCE A BIT OF LOW-FRUCTOSE FRUIT AND TO MAKE MY TREATS WITH AS LITTLE SWEETENER AS POSSIBLE.

Look out for this little icon in the recipe section. It denotes sweet-free recipes suitable for quitting and recalibrating.

8WP

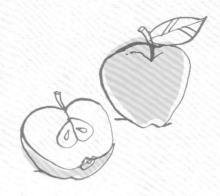

READ YOUR LABELS

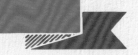

STEP 5

Allow for bigger serving sizes: double the amount if you have to.

I personally eat more than an average serve of most foods. You too? Check out how many serves there are in a packet and round your figure up if you're eating more than the suggested serving size.

NUTRITION INFORMATION
SERVINGS PER PACKAGE 3.2   SERVING SIZE 170 g

	Ave Quantity per Serving	Ave Quantity per 100 g
Energy	697 kJ (167 Cal)	410 kJ (98 Cal)
Protein – total	9.1 g	5.3 g
– gluten	0 mg	0 mg
Fat – total	2.7 g	1.6 g
– saturated	1.7 g	1.0 g
Carbohydrate total	26.2 g	15.4 g
Sugars	25.7 g	15.1 g
Sodium	135 mg	79 mg
Calcium	295 mg (37%RDI)	173 mg

LOW-FAT YOGHURT

STEP 1

A quick snapshot: choose foods with less than 5 g of sugar/100 g, or 5% sugar.

This quick reading should keep you roughly in check and will wipe out 90% of processed foods. This low-fat yoghurt is 15% sugar.

STEP 2

But if it's dairy remember the first 4.7 g of sugar/100 g is lactose.

Lactose is fine to consume, but anything on top of the 4.7 g is added sugar. Here, the amount of added sugar/100 g is 10.4 g. (15.1 g average quantity of sugar per 100 g minus 4.7 g.) This is the amount you work with in your calculations.

STEP 4

To calculate the sugar content in teaspoons, divide the sugar content by 4.2.

So 4.2 g of sugar = 1 teaspoon; 8.4 g = 2 teaspoons. Work out how much you're eating in a serve by dividing the serving size by roughly 4 to get an idea of how much you're eating. I find it easier to visualise amounts in teaspoons. You too?

Here we take the 25.7 g (or 17.7 g if you want to take the lactose-free figure) and divide it by 4.2. Thus, 6.1 teaspoons of sugar per serve, or 4.2 teaspoons lactose-free.

STEP 3

And if it's a liquid: it must contain no sugar.

A serving size for a juice can be 375 ml, some servings can be up to 750 ml (at those juice bars). Pasta sauce can be 250 ml, which means the per 100 ml quantity of sugar needs to be multiplied by about a factor of 4, 7.5 and 2.5 (respectively) to work out how much sugar it actually contains. Even if it's only 5% sugar, a liquid's massive serving size renders it a sugary dump. Here, for instance, you need to multiply the 10.4 g (see step 2) by a factor of 1.7 as you're not eating 100 g. You're eating 170 g. That's 17.7 g in the one serve.

The take-home: never drink anything containing sugar!

REMEMBER: It's recommended we consume no more than 5–9 teaspoons of sugar a day.

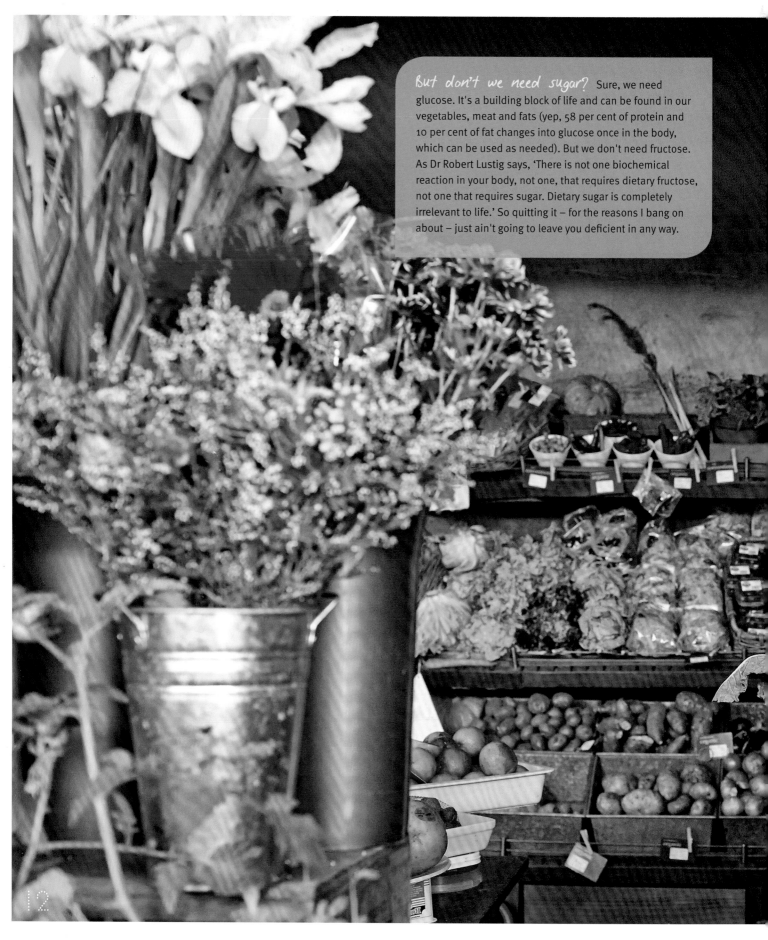

But don't we need sugar? Sure, we need glucose. It's a building block of life and can be found in our vegetables, meat and fats (yep, 58 per cent of protein and 10 per cent of fat changes into glucose once in the body, which can be used as needed). But we don't need fructose. As Dr Robert Lustig says, 'There is not one biochemical reaction in your body, not one, that requires dietary fructose, not one that requires sugar. Dietary sugar is completely irrelevant to life.' So quitting it – for the reasons I bang on about – just ain't going to leave you deficient in any way.

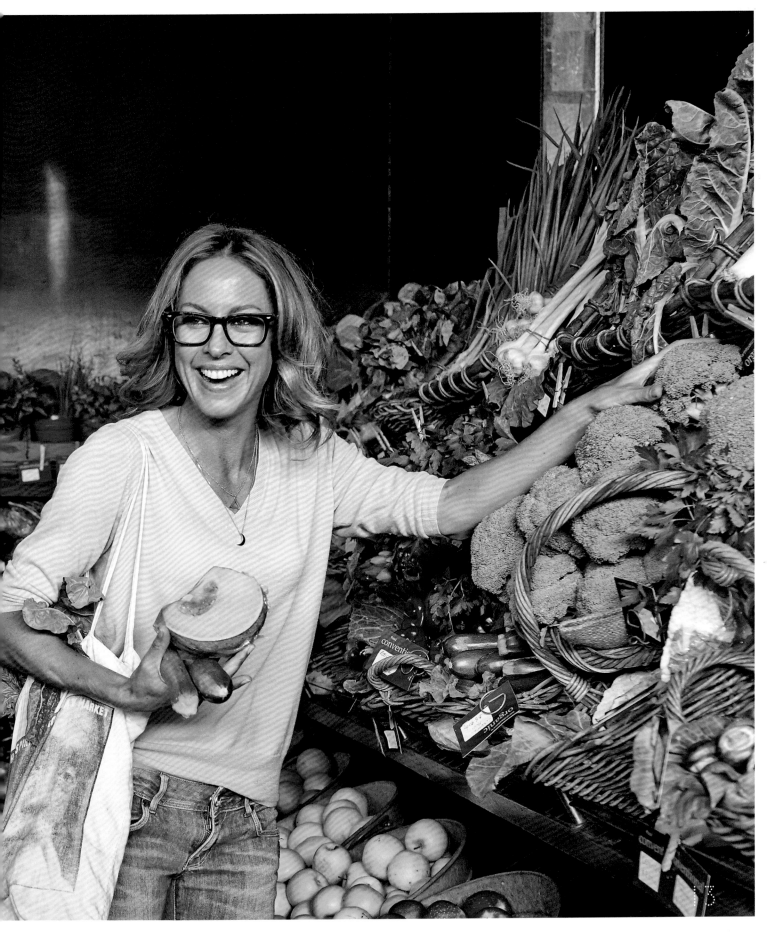

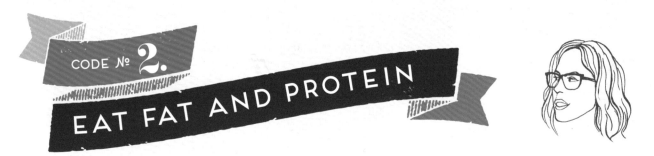

EAT FAT AND PROTEIN

THE SECRET INGREDIENT TO QUITTING SUGAR FOR LIFE IS EATING MORE FAT AND PROTEIN, which will get your body rebalanced and burning the right kind of fuel. It will also nip blood sugar dips and see you eat less – and less often. And very possibly lose weight.

TO RECAP FROM LAST TIME:

Fat fills us up.

Fats (and protein) have corresponding hormones that coordinate with our brain to switch off our appetite when we've eaten enough. Fructose has no such corresponding 'off-switch' hormone, and so we can keep eating and eating it. Which is why we can drink 750 ml of apple juice or soft drink; try drinking that much full-fat yoghurt. Actually, don't; it's impossible!

THROW A LOG ON THE FIRE.

My dear friend Nora Gedgaudas, author of *Primal Body, Primal Mind*, once explained the beauty of fat and protein thus: 'When you eat sugar, it's like throwing paper or kerosene on your metabolic fire. Sure it will burn, but you'll have to continuously throw more on to stop the flame dying out. Fat and protein, on the other hand is like a solid log to the fire. It will burn slowly and evenly for a good four to six hours before needing to be replaced.'

Fat isn't addictive.

Fructose is; indeed, studies show it's more addictive than cocaine and heroin.

Fat is burnt as fuel, not stored as fat.

Fructose, however, is mostly processed in the liver. The liver doesn't recognise it as a valid foodstuff, gets confused and stores it as triglycerides, which are bad fats (the short story).

We're designed to get fat on sugar.

This fact brings me comfort. It means our bodies are doing what they're meant to be doing, and nothing is amiss. Back in caveman days, when sugar was so very rare, it was evolutionarily advantageous to get fat from sugar. Fat meant survival. It was therefore also advantageous to have no fructose on/off switch, so that when we did stumble upon a rare berry bush or beehive, we could binge on it and stock up on fat reserves. All this also explains why sugar is addictive – again, it was evolutionarily advantageous to be obsessed with sugar – so we could get fat on it.

SUGAR IS NATURAL. GETTING FAT ON SUGAR IS NATURAL. LET'S THINK ABOUT THAT FOR A MINUTE.

THE AMOUNT OF SUGAR WE NOW EAT, HOWEVER, IS NOT NATURAL.

Fat fuels our metabolism.

Indeed it's actually required to activate metabolism and to absorb essential vitamins A, E, D and K from the vegetables and fruits we eat. Eating (good) fat can actually help you lose weight. Fact.

BUT WHAT ABOUT CHOLESTEROL? WHAT ABOUT HEART DISEASE?

I'll put it simply. Cholesterol (bad, good, HDL, LDL, whatever) is a sticking plaster (as well as being a critical molecule for hormone health and more). It circulates in our arteries, patching up damage caused by the damage that sugar – yes, sugar – and other toxins cause. Cholesterol ain't the problem. It's the fix. Further, studies show saturated fat intake doesn't raise blood cholesterol levels. And *even* further, there's zero evidence that eating high-cholesterol foods causes heart disease. In fact, many argue that the vegetable oils and margarine we've been told to eat instead are the culprits. Read more on this via the interweb if you have cholesterol issues!

EAT THE RIGHT FATS To continue sugar-free successfully for life, you need to switch from being a sugar-burning machine to a fat-burning one (logs instead of kerosene). But this is not a licence to eat fries and corn chips. Only some fats are good. And most need to be eaten in particular ways:

Pour or dollop (cold) with: Saturated fats (butter) and mono-unsaturated fats (olive oil and nut oils like macadamia or avocado) are great. Even at room temperature the poly-unsaturateds (the so-called vegetable oils like rapeseed, soya bean and sunflower) are problematic because once in our warm bodies they heat up and become unstable.

Sauté with: Again, any saturated and most mono-unsaturated and nut oils are great at medium temperatures. The vegetable oils should never be heated – they're unstable and at high temperatures they oxidise, leading to inflammation.

STOP 'FRYING' YOUR VEGETABLES Most everyday fats, even butter and olive oil, should only be cooked to medium–high temperatures. When fried at super-hot temperatures they, too, become unstable – and oxidise. Instead 'sweat' them *slowly* at a lower temperature. Take a good 15 minutes with your onions, for instance. This is how the long-living folk in the Mediterranean cook their vegetables. They know that pushing the heat higher renders the oils unhealthy. Slow and low also best precipitates the Maillard and caramelisation reactions that provide the luscious sweet flavours from meats and vegetables.

Fry (if you must) with: ghee and coconut oil. Or lard if you have it. My favourites: I fry chicken, 'sweet' vegetables (like pumpkin) and foods (like curry) in coconut oil. I use ghee for most other frying and olive oil occasionally (where I can keep the heat a little below a robust fry).

Don't touch (ever): poly-unsaturated oils (rapeseed, soya bean, sunflower). I also advise against consuming omega-3 oils. Even with small temperature fluctuations, they can turn unstable (and convert into the unhealthy omega-6); eat fish instead.

EAT *MORE* FAT I find those who don't up their *good* fat content generally struggle to get results on the IQS programme. Their cravings aren't curbed, they're not maximising their nutrition and they don't lose weight. What I'm suggesting isn't about getting all Atkins-extreme and eating bacon-wrapped sausages every other meal. It's about sensible, nutritious tweaks:

▶ Add: ½ tablespoon per person of butter, coconut oil, extra-virgin olive oil, macadamia or avocado oil to steamed vegetables and salads.

▶ Remember: Vegetables should always be eaten with fat so that the important vitamins A, E, K and D, which are fat-soluble only, can work their magic.

▶ *Also* add: 1–2 tablespoons per person of avocado, nuts, seeds or cheese to vegetables and salads, wherever possible.

▶ Eat the whole food. That is, the skin on pork and chicken, egg yolks (with the whites) and full-fat milk (never skimmed). Food is designed to be consumed as a whole package and becomes less nutritious when tampered with. Egg yolks, for instance, contain the enzymes that help us metabolise the egg as a whole. And when you remove the fat from dairy, much of the enzyme lactase is also taken out, rendering the milk less digestible and ultimately more fattening. Indeed!

Q. WHAT IF I'M EATING TOO MUCH FAT?

Simple answer: don't worry, you're probably not, so long as you're eating the right fats. Your body is beautifully tuned to turn you off fat when you've eaten enough. When we first switch to this way of eating, some of us can have a tendency to go a little too hard on the fat and it can take a few weeks for the body to adjust and find the right balance. If you're concerned you're possibly over-doing it, here's a trick: halve your fat of choice, say, a serve of cheese, after dinner. Wait 10 minutes after eating the first half and see what your body says. If it's had enough, you'll know. If not, enjoy that other half!

What's the FUSS with COCONUT OIL?

Coconut oil is mostly made up of medium-chain fatty acids (MCFAs), which permeate cell membranes easily, do not require special enzymes to be utilised effectively by your body, and put minimal strain on your digestive system.

These factors, and more, imbue coconut oil with a bunch of unique health benefits:

▶ **It helps you lose weight.** MCFAs are sent directly to your liver, where they're immediately converted into energy rather than being stored as fat. This promotes 'thermogenesis' (the 'burning up' of your food), which increases the body's metabolism, leading to weight loss.

▶ **It curbs slumps and cravings.** Both carbs and coconut oil deliver quick energy to your body, but the latter doesn't produce an insulin spike in your bloodstream, while the former does.

▶ **It's the healthiest oil to cook with.** Which I've already had a chat about.

▶ **It's anti-viral and anti-fungal.** A 'miracle' fat called lauric acid makes up 50% of the fat in coconut oil. Interestingly, the only other place it can be found is breast milk. Your body converts lauric acid into monolaurin, which has anti-viral, antibacterial and anti-protozoal properties. This means that coconut oil is also great for controlling candida (thrush), which is caused by a fungus.

▶ **It's anti-inflammatory.** There are many advantages to boosting your metabolic rate: your body's healing process accelerates, cell regeneration increases to replace old cells, and your immune system works better overall. When your immune system is functioning well, your body will be less inflamed.

▶ **It's REALLY good for thyroid issues.** Coconut oil can also raise basal body temperatures while increasing metabolism. This is good news for people who suffer with low thyroid function. *Like me.*

▶▶▶ LET'S TRY THIS ◀◀◀
EAT A SPOONFUL OF COCONUT OIL AFTER LUNCH

My number-one, hands-down, foolproof way to curb cravings is to:

▶ Grab a jar of 100% organic, raw and virgin coconut oil.

▶ Scoop out 1 heaped tablespoon.
(Option: mix with ⅓ teaspoon of raw cacao powder.)

▶ Eat as you would a scoop of mousse.

▶ Wait 5–8 minutes (walk around the block, hang out the washing, make a phone call).

▶ Now reflect on how satiated you feel, and how the sweet cravings have gone.

Eating it after lunch will nip that 'Now I need something sweet' hankering in its tiresome bud and keep you fighting full until dinner.

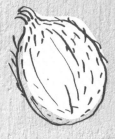
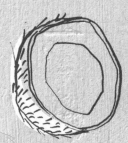

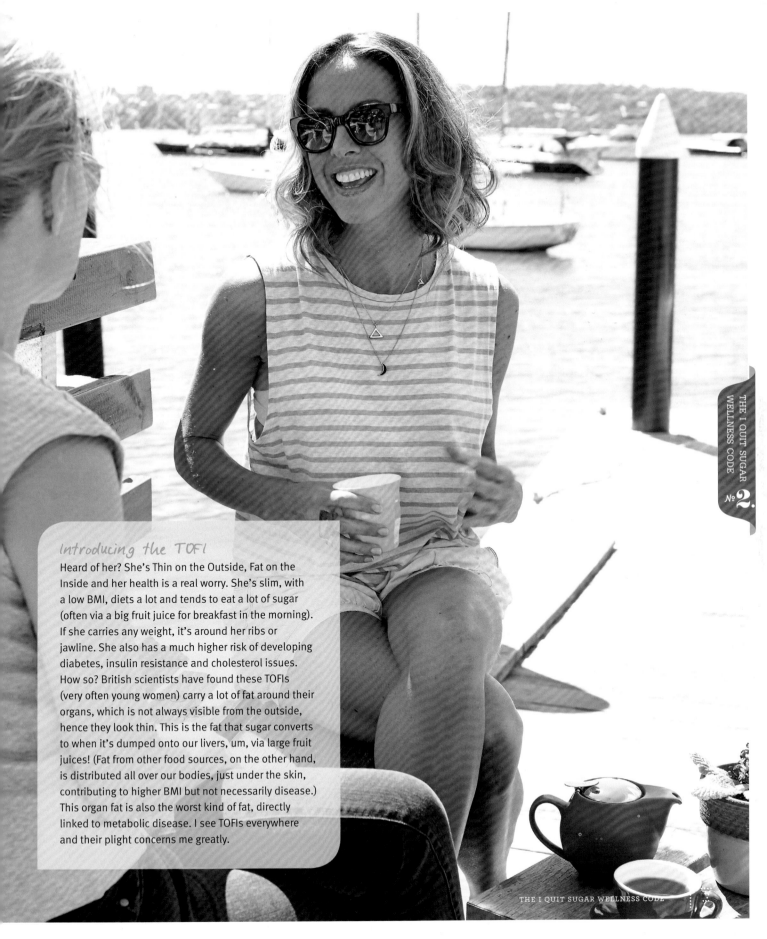

Introducing the TOFI

Heard of her? She's Thin on the Outside, Fat on the Inside and her health is a real worry. She's slim, with a low BMI, diets a lot and tends to eat a lot of sugar (often via a big fruit juice for breakfast in the morning). If she carries any weight, it's around her ribs or jawline. She also has a much higher risk of developing diabetes, insulin resistance and cholesterol issues. How so? British scientists have found these TOFIs (very often young women) carry a lot of fat around their organs, which is not always visible from the outside, hence they look thin. This is the fat that sugar converts to when it's dumped onto our livers, um, via large fruit juices! (Fat from other food sources, on the other hand, is distributed all over our bodies, just under the skin, contributing to higher BMI but not necessarily disease.) This organ fat is also the worst kind of fat, directly linked to metabolic disease. I see TOFIs everywhere and their plight concerns me greatly.

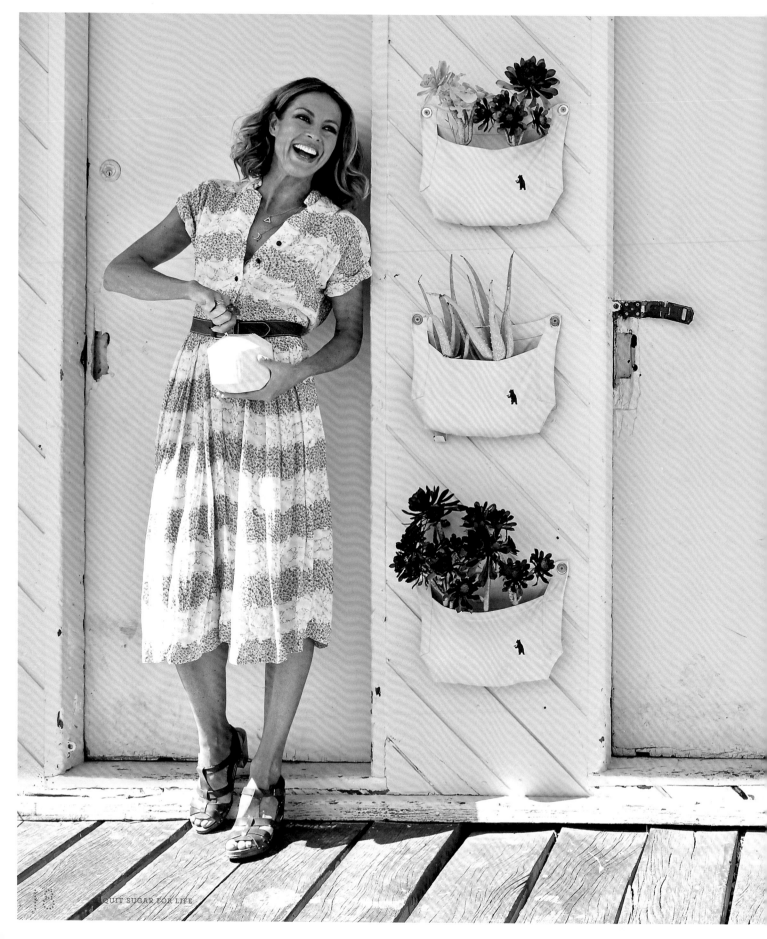

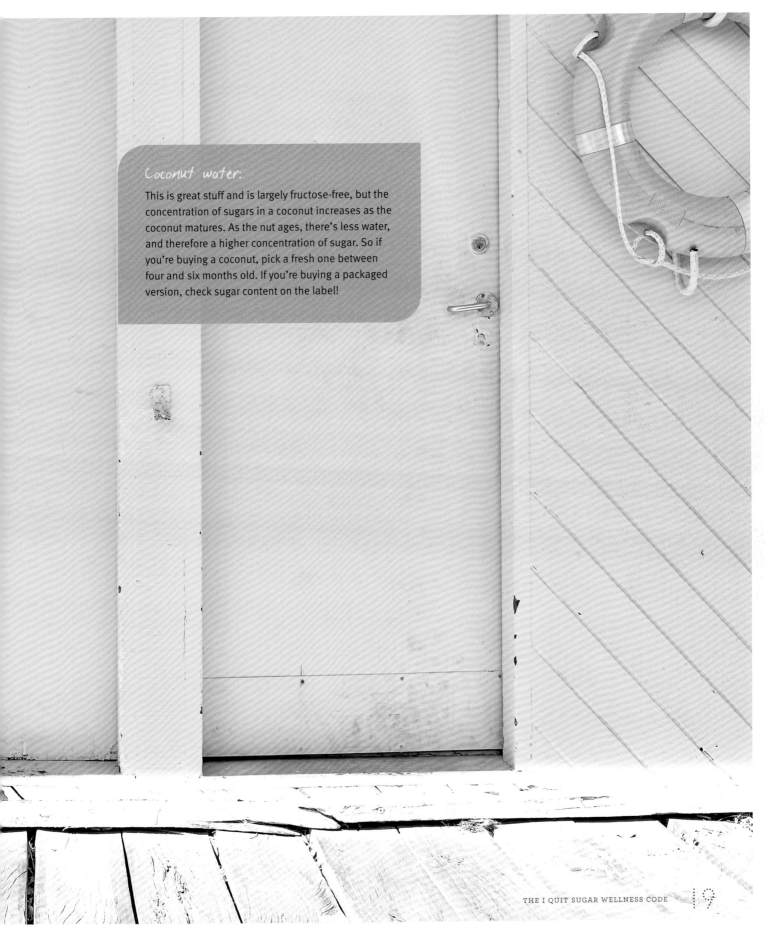

Coconut water:

This is great stuff and is largely fructose-free, but the concentration of sugars in a coconut increases as the coconut matures. As the nut ages, there's less water, and therefore a higher concentration of sugar. So if you're buying a coconut, pick a fresh one between four and six months old. If you're buying a packaged version, check sugar content on the label!

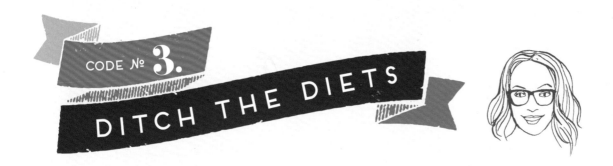

DIETS DON'T WORK. PERIOD. TRUE WELLNESS IS ABOUT BEING FREE FROM RESTRICTION AND EXTREMES. That said, some diets can have some valid nutritional principles at their core. True wellness is also about being open and cherrypicking helpful tips and tricks, and seeing if it works for you.

This is the boon of living without sugar – it gets your body off the sugar rollercoaster and able to determine the eating approaches that best suit you.

Know this: there is no perfect diet or eating approach. None are scientifically 'proven', including the sugar-free one. It's all an experiment. Let's check out a bunch of dietary ideas that you might be able to cherrypick the best of:

CLEANSING, DETOXING AND JUICING

Juice cleanses, lemon juice and cayenne fasts, coffee enema retreats . . . the idea is that by flushing everything out and getting nutrients in an easily digestible (mostly liquid) form we can get our bodies back on the straight and narrow. But here's the funny thing: the body is already plenty capable of eliminating toxins on its own. And daily. It's called, ah, urination. Also . . .

OUR BODIES DETOX BEST WITH – WAIT FOR IT – SUGAR-FREE FOOD.

There's also this: liquid diets leave you hungry (solids take almost twice as long as liquids to leave your stomach) and constipated (you need fibre for your gut to move and to maintain the right kind of bacteria to keep things active), and will slow your metabolism (the calorie decrease can send the body into starvation mode, causing you to store

energy). Plus, juices are often full of fruit, beetroot and carrot, which, when the fibre is removed, are instant sugary fat dumps to the liver, served in a cute bottle.

There are certainly benefits to resting your digestion from time to time. But I have some simpler, smarter suggestions.

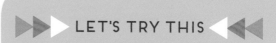

LET'S TRY THIS

VEGETABLE SMOOTHIES INSTEAD OF JUICES

Liquefying your meals can have benefits – it can be quite soothing and can give your digestion a break. But puréeing instead of juicing your vegetables is a far better way to go. You retain the fibre (and extra nutrients in the skin) and it can also help you metabolise any sugar content. Eat/drink a Green Glowin' Skin Smoothie for breakfast each morning for a week, with some fat (avocado, nuts, coconut oil), and you'll be flushingly clean in no time.

FASTING

I don't like the idea of food deprivation for days on end – it's too emotionally taxing for most of us. But I can see the benefit of giving your guts a good rest in regular spurts, and intermittent fasts, such as the 5:2 and the Alternate Day Fast, are backed by some sound science and logic. Clinical trials show that reduced caloric intake a few days a week reduces circulating sugar and fat levels and reduces blood pressure, inflammation and oxidative stress. Research at the US National Institute on Aging's neuroscience laboratory suggests fasting is a mild form of stress that stimulates the body's cellular defences against molecular damage, thus improving longevity. Other studies show a 14–16-hour food break can have similar benefits. This gels with me as it's easily done, even daily.

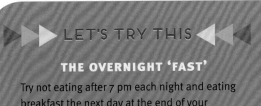

►► LET'S TRY THIS ◄◄

THE OVERNIGHT 'FAST'

Try not eating after 7 pm each night and eating breakfast the next day at the end of your morning routine (see Code 5). Whaddya know? You have yourself a daily 14-hour fast. I find this approach is quite effective for setting my appetite for the day. Only try this technique if you're curious or if you feel your digestion might be over-taxed, of course.

BEWARE

PROCESSED FOODS CONTAIN EXTRA CALORIES DER, RIGHT? A RECENT STUDY FOUND THAT IF YOU EAT A 600-CALORIE SERVING OF WHOLE-MEAL BREAD WITH REAL CHEESE, YOU EXPEND TWICE AS MUCH ENERGY DIGESTING IT THAN IF YOU EAT 600 CALORIES OF WHITE BREAD WITH PROCESSED CHEESE. REAL FOOD – IT'S A HEALTHY WORKOUT!

RAW FOODISM

Fans of this approach maintain that cooking reduces a *food's* enzymes and the fewer enzymes in a food, the more our own *body's* enzymes must be drawn upon to break down a meal. The more of our own enzymes we use, the quicker we age . . . Got it?

Sure, some uncooked food in our diet, daily, is a good thing. However, many of the vitamins and minerals in vegetables are embedded in the plant's cellulose cell walls, which require cooking to break them down. So many of the valuable nutrients in raw vegetables end up not being absorbed by the body. Also, 'raw food' products often contain a ton of agave and coconut sugar, with the sell-in that it's raw. Yeah, raw, but toxic. So, what to do?

►► LET'S TRY THIS ◄◄

NOT BLASTING THE CRAP OUT OF OUR FOOD

There's a middle ground here – we can preserve enzymes *and* access vitamins and minerals by cooking our food slow and low.

▶ **'Sweat'** your vegetables gently at a low heat instead of stir-frying. I've touched on this already.

▶ **Slow-cook** your meat and legumes instead of frying or boiling them. Many of the recipes in this book use this method, as you'll soon learn.

ADDING A DASH OF RAW

Eating a combination of cooked vegetables with some raw stuff is a great idea.

▶ In summer, eat a salad regularly. In winter, bear in mind winter vegetables are rarely suited to eating as a salad so instead, try adding to your steamed vegetables or cooked meals some chopped raw carrot or red onion or – best option – some fermented vegetables (see page 198). I like to stir a tablespoon or two through my Midweek One-Pot Meals (see page 109). The activated enzymes in cultured food overcomes the 'tough cell' issue I mentioned.

GLUTEN-FREE EATING

If you have a gluten intolerance, coeliac disease or, indeed, any kind of auto-immune disease, you know not to touch even a speck of gluten, right? Even a speck will remain in your system for six months and wreak havoc. For everyone else on the planet, sensitive or otherwise? Well, gluten contains toxins. These toxins are wheat's only defence against predators (us). Plus, products today contain way more gluten than they did even just 20 years ago. Further, we're eating more of it today than ever before (on average 6–8 servings a day). Ergo, we're consuming increasing quantities of a toxin that causes digestion issues and inflammation, and leaches valuable minerals from our bodies. Add all this together and you can probably see why gluten is causing so many health issues.

I believe it's a good idea to take charge and limit your gluten where you can.

RECIPE TO TRY

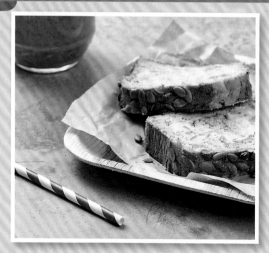

PALEO INSIDE-OUT BREAD:

This is a fun gluten-free bread idea and a complete meal in itself (see page 61).

PALEO DIET

Heard of it? Perhaps you know it as the 'caveman diet'. The premise is that eating as our forebears used to, before the advent of agriculture 10,000 years ago, serves us best. This period is roughly when our genes and metabolic processes developed. With agriculture came a whole bunch of foods we struggle to consume – primarily grains and legumes – and that also compromise the ecosystem. Our diets have changed radically, but our genes and metabolism have not, goes the argument.

The paleo approach is fundamentally low-starch, anti-processed and pro-organic. It turns to meat (pasture-fed; nose-to-tail cuts), saturated fats (no processed or seed oils) and vegetables, with a little fruit. Some paleo types eat eggs, dairy and nuts and some starches such as sweet potato. Some don't. Paleo is also anti-sugar, and the philosophy overall – eating whole, living sustainably and dodging toxins and stressors – is on the same page as what I'm banging on about here.

If you're PALEO or GLUTEN-FREE . . .

The recipes in this book are largely gluten- and grain-free, simply to cut down on toxic load, but also because when you go sugar-free, it necessarily eliminates a lot of processed carbs anyway. Where a gluten or grain product is used, it's easy to substitute the following options:

▶ courgette 'pasta' (see page 106)

▶ gluten-free pasta

▶ quinoa (see page 94), millet, amaranth or buckwheat (all of which are seeds, not grains)

▶ gluten-free and nut flours (be sure to add extra butter or oil when using nut flours)

▶ coconut flour (but add extra liquid)

▶ rice – jasmine and basmati are best: they're not as high in the grain fibres that cause so many gut issues. Brown rice contains a lot of phytic acid.

▶ extra vegetables – a whole baked sweet potato is a good choice. (Simply place the whole sweet potato, skin and all, on a baking tray and roast in the oven – preheated to 200°C (gas 6) – for 45 minutes or until tender.)

CUT CARBS FOR TWO WEEKS

(If you've been off sugar for some time)

If you're curious about whether carb-less living might do good stuff for you, cut back on, or cut out, bread, wraps, pasta, rice, cereal, pizza, noodles, polenta, etc. and see how it makes *you* feel. Replace them with the substitutes in the box on the left. Keep a food diary, or at least get mindful of any reactions, shifts in energy, cravings, gut issues and weight changes. And slowly reintroduce carbs back in if you're just not feeling great. I also advise doing this experiment alongside a doctor or nutrition professional who can monitor your health with blood testing before and during. Also: if you have compromised health, please research this issue further and consult a nutritionist or doctor before jumping in. Abruptly cutting all carbs can cause weight fluctuations and related hormonal issues.

 WHICH BREAD SHOULD I EAT, SUGAR-WISE?

If you're not gluten intolerant, genuine sourdough is best. The cultures in the sourdough partially break down gluten and slow our absorption of the sugars in white flour, plus they activate the enzymes required to break down the phytic acid. Even commercial sourdoughs contain less sugar than most other breads.

 SHOULD I QUIT CARBS WHEN I QUIT SUGAR?

A good question. Three points:

1. One thing at a time. I don't advise quitting both sugar and carbs at the same time. It's too much denial and change in one hit.

2. Experiment. Some people do find after quitting sugar for some time that their tolerance for carbs is lessened and that grains and starches, particularly refined ones, keep them in a cycle of blood sugar ups and downs and cravings. Cutting (back on) carbs helps these people. In the past decade, more than 20 randomised controlled trials have shown low-carb diets are effective in reducing blood pressure, weight gain, cholesterol problems, blood sugar issues and that it's an easier dietary approach to stick to than, say, low-fat diets.

3. Overall, though, I reckon it's best to avoid refined carbs. They're redundant calories and get in the way of denser nutrition. It's also good to limit gluten-containing foods, as well as legumes, due to the toxic load they place on our bodies.

THE I QUIT SUGAR WELLNESS CODE № 3.

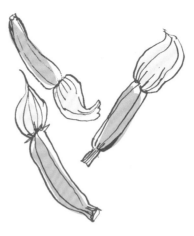

CALORIE-COUNTING

Please know this: calorie-counting is a waste of energy. How so? It doesn't take into account the *way* we burn energy once the food is in our gob. We are *not* 'calorie-in-calorie-out' machines, despite what some antiquated diet pedlars like to claim. We're more complex than that. For instance, starchy, fibrous veggies contain a lot fewer calories once they're inside us – we burn more energy accessing the calories through the hard-to-rupture cell walls. Further, cooking ruptures most cell walls, so cooked veggies have more calories than raw. And what about this: once digested, protein foods contain fewer calories than are listed on the label.

How so? Again, because it takes a lot of energy to break the protein down. Plus, some proteins require our immune system to get involved during digestion, which burns even more calories.

VEGANISM

Can I be frank here? My research has led me to conclude that a meat-inclusive diet is more ethical, more environmentally sustainable and more nutritious per calorie intake than a grain- and legume-based one. In Australia, 22 times more animals are killed to produce the latter, through destruction of habitat to make room for agriculture. That said, I'm grateful to vegans for placing the issue on the table. Every meat-eater should be made aware of these issues and eat meat mindfully (see 'Shop Differently' on page 42). Plus this much we all agree on: vegetables are the bomb. For more reading on this subject – and I really do encourage it on this important topic – see the 'Reading List' on page 226.

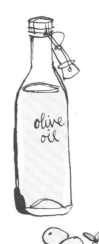

If you're VEGAN, VEGETARIAN or EAT DAIRY-FREE . . .

Many of the recipes in this book contain eggs, dairy and meat. However, you can make your own substitutions according to your needs, but please be mindful of a few things (I consulted my vegan mate Sarah from MyNewRoots.org on this one):

▶ Only use grains, legumes and nuts that have been soaked and activated (see page 204), fermented (see page 197) or sprouted (see page 162). These practices minimise phytic acid, a toxin that leaches valuable minerals from our bodies and damages the gut lining, leading to 'leaky gut' and a host of resulting health issues from there.

▶ Avoid soya products in general, unless they've been fermented (miso and tempeh), and even then only in small amounts, for similar reasons as above.

▶ Beware: many packaged vegan foods are highly processed and packed with sugar and chemicals.

▶ Take *extra* care to ensure you get enough fat and protein at every meal. Dose up by adding to meals:

    *a vegan protein powder (these are processed and not the most ideal way to ingest protein, but a good stop-gap)

    *chia seeds (which contain 18 amino acids and are 23% protein)

    *coconut products

    *oils: macadamia, avocado, coconut, olive.

    *also try: whole hulled hemp seeds / hearts and hemp products (oil, ground powder), spirulina and chlorella.

▶ Choose substitute milks with the lowest amount of sugar. Some use rice malt syrup instead of sugar; invest in these. Or make your own nut milk (there's a recipe in *I Quit Sugar*).

▶ Make nutritionally sound swaps:

    *cheese — avocado or nutritional yeast
    *butter — coconut oil
    *meat — mushrooms and sprouted brown lentils
    *slow-cooked meat — spaghetti squash
    *eggs (for binding) — 1 tablespoon chia seeds (ground) mixed with 3 tablespoons water per egg

How do you DEAL with LAPSES?

Well, first, I don't freak. Quitting sugar for life simply means making the best available wellness choices and doing your best (by yourself). It's a gentle, curious experiment, not a mean diet. Also, this: so-called lapses are good! They are perfect for reminding us why we choose not to eat sugar.

Take comfort: once you know the deal with sugar, you don't go back to where you started. 'You can't unlearn this stuff!'

When I do get too far outta whack, however – like when my sugar intake creeps up or when I've been eating out too much, drinking coffee daily, not getting enough sleep – I recalibrate. I do a mini 8-week programme, just for a few days.

And here's the thing about recalibrating: this gentle steering back to the 'blank slate' is precisely what instils stronger habits.

I recalibrate by:

- Eating extra protein and fat
- Drinking an extra litre of water a day
- Drinking no alcohol or stimulants (so I can give the liver a rest; green tea is OK)
- Doing my coconut oil after lunch trick
- Obviously not eating any sugar, nor sweetener (including stevia and rice malt syrup and fruit)
- Pacifying my Vata (see page 26) by eating lots of warm, smooth foods, for example
- Sweating – via exercise, hot yoga and infra-red sauna
- Having a green smoothie each morning and adding extra greens at every other meal.

And if I'm really wanting to reset right, I do a 'Clean Week', eating super dense nutrition for 5 days (yeah, I know, not quite a week!).

THE BEST DIET: AYURVEDA!

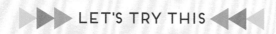

An Indian approach dating back 5000 years (Buddhism stemmed from the tradition 2000 years later), Ayurveda's central thread is balance. You don't fix health issues; you heal with balance. I like this. No, I love it. Living sugar-free for life is about balance and finding your own through food and energy restoration. This Wellness Code incorporates a lot of Ayurvedic philosophy and practices. Not surprising since I've been working with it for a few years now.

Never heard of Ayurveda? Let me flesh out a little. The tradition (to which Deepak Chopra, the Beatles and David Lynch have all been subscribers) incorporates diet as well as other lifestyle habits and works to three doshas, or body types. Each of us is a combination of all three types, but tend to have one that dominates. Wellness is about ensuring our dominant dosha (in my case it's Vata) is happy and balanced, not aggravated or too dominant. We do this with a bit of gentle recalibration and tweaking; no dieting, just some supplementing.

IF YOU'RE PREDOMINANTLY VATA, you tend to be thin, tall, light and quick in your thoughts and actions. Change is a constant part of your life. You're FLIGHTY! Vatas *hate* the cold and love summer and can have very dry hair and skin.

When you're in balance, you are creative, enthusiastic, chatty and lively. But if Vata becomes excessive, you may develop anxiety, insomnia, constipation, irregular digestion, dizziness and disjointed thoughts.

How to balance Vata: Calm down! Do this with warm, soft, cooked, oily and grounding foods (stews, fats, root vegetables, ginger and other 'chai-like' spices). Berries, 'sweet' foods like sweet potato and dairy are good, but avoid stimulants (back away from the coffee!) and cold salads. Facial and body oils are great (I love roseship oil on my face and coconut or sesame oil on my body), so is eating extra oil. It's best to maintain regular habits (eat and sleep at the same times), rest, stay out of the wind and away from air-con and to exercise gently – yoga, swimming, a bit of weights and walking are best, even though you have a natural tendency to want to do frenetic cardio. Oh, and make friends with a balanced Kapha type – they're lovely and grounding for a Vata.

RECIPE TO TRY

If you're VATA

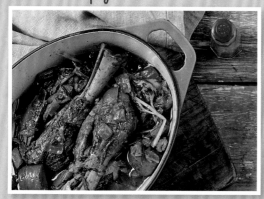

LEMON AND CINNAMON LAMB SHANKS WITH GREMOLATA

A GREAT VATA BALANCER (see page 119): warm, soft and grounding

BE VATA-AWARE

Many of us in the West tend to be Vata-dominant. Our culture almost demands it! What's more, whatever your dominant type, if your Vata is wobbly – frenetic, over-stimulated (from eating too much sugar!) and anxious – the other doshas will also become unbalanced. And so keeping Vata happy is the key to good health.

A few things to keep an eye out for, which will render you imbalanced no matter your type: air-conditioning, plane travel, noisy city life, frenetic schedules and frantic exercise.

IF YOU'RE PREDOMINANTLY PITTA, you're muscular, medium-build, often with a reddish complexion and freckles (both light ones and dark spots). Your force is fire – so summer throws a Pitta person right outta whack and you can sweat . . . a lot!

When balanced, you are warm, intelligent, focused and determined and a great leader.

If out of balance, Pitta types can be judgemental, irritable and aggressive. They get 'hot' symptoms, such as heartburn, burning eyes, acne and acid stomach. I've noticed Pitta men are often bald (too much heat coming out the top of their heads!).

How to balance Pitta: Cool down! Eat salad-y and watery foods such as coriander, avocado, cucumber and dark, leafy greens (kale, baby spinach leaves) and avoid fried or spicy foods. Keep out of the sun and surround yourself with cooling colours. Do not go near a hot yoga class (Bikram ain't your friend!); water sports are perfect. You tend to like aggressive, competitive sports – back off from these when you're hot and Pitta-ish and try yoga, walking and more graceful pursuits.

IF YOU'RE PREDOMINANTLY KAPHA, you have a strong and large body frame; thick, curly hair; and thick, smooth, oily and hairy skin.

In balance, you are calm, steady and patient, sleep well, have perfect digestion and enjoy life without worry. You're pretty laid-back.

When out of balance, your digestion can be slow, and you can be prone to weight gain, fluid retention, allergies, depression and excessive sleep. Kapha is an earthy dosha and can make you heavy and stagnant – you need firing up!

How to balance Kapha: Choose foods that are light, sprightly and spicy. Ginger, black pepper, cumin, chilli and lots of bitter dark greens are your friends. Coffee can be good when you're a bit heavily Kaphic, to get you motivated. Avoid heavy oily foods and, yes, sugar. You have great stamina and strength, but when you're out of whack (and sluggish), cardio is best. Also, you might like to surround yourself with a Vata type – their energy will help to motivate you out of the slump.

RECIPE TO TRY

If you're PITTA

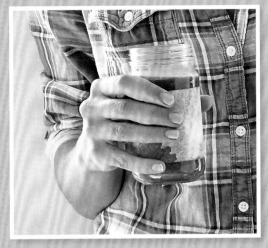

I AM GRACEFUL (ANTI-INFLAMMATORY BLEND) GREEN GLOWIN' SKIN SMOOTHIE (see page 77)

RECIPE TO TRY

If you're KAPHA

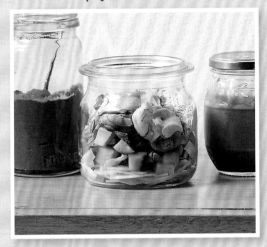

PRAWN COCKTAIL MISH-MASH GREAT GRATED SALAD (see page 83)

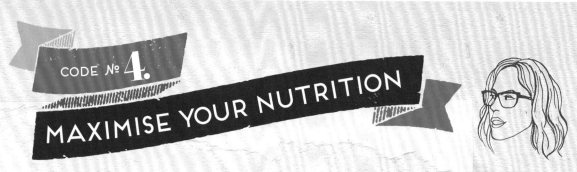

MAXIMISE YOUR NUTRITION

OK. IF YOU'VE JUST DIGESTED CODE #3, YOUR HEAD MIGHT BE SPINNING FROM ALL THE COMPETING MESSAGES. I get it. If this is you, feel free to shelve the whole lot and cut to the culinary chase with a far more elegant edict, which I use to guide myself in my sugar-free life …

This is the guiding philosophy to my eating.

IQS MANTRA 5.

EAT DENSE At every opportunity eat foods with the densest nutrition.

Eating dense is not difficult. It's mostly about adding to what you do, thus:
▶ prioritising (and adding extra) leafy greens and high-quality fat and protein at every meal.
▶ preparing food to preserve (and maximise) enzymes and bacteria for digestion.
▶ eliminating toxins and empty calories (um, sugar).

Get dense and everything else – detoxing, fuelling, dealing with sugar swings and staying slim – is taken care of.

So how do I do this? I employ some dense eating tricks.

These ideas also happen to be economical, efficient and environmental-friendly, too:

▶ **Always add fat to your vegetables** so that you can properly absorb the essential vitamins A, E, D and K. I know I'm repeating myself, but it's an important shift to be made.

▶ **Ditto, always eat fat with protein.** Fat is needed for proper protein assimilation. Never eat an egg white omelette and don't pick the skin off your chook or roast pork!

▶ **Prioritise your veg.** All vegetables are your friends, but if you want to up the ante, eat leafy greens (the most nutritious option) over other greens over starchy vegetables.

▶ **Eat more protein**. Our skin, bones, hair and nails are mostly made up of protein. The best sources of proteins are dairy, eggs, meat and fish – because animal protein is complete, it contains the right proportions of all the essential amino acids our bodies can't synthesise on their own. Proteins offer the most energy per caloric intake of all foods.

▶ **Eat 'tough' meat cuts, such as beef chuck, osso bucco, pork neck and lamb shanks.** They come from muscles on the animal that contain the greatest amount of connective tissue, which – when slow-cooked – dissolves into gelatine. Gelatine not only aids digestion, it repairs the integrity of a damaged gut.

▶ **Eat chicken drumsticks.** The dark meat of chicken contains more minerals than the white. And – boon! – it's cheaper.

▶ **Actually, eat the whole chook.** The greatest bang comes from eating the meat as well as the carcass, boiled up as a stock. The bones, skin and giblets contain the life-giving minerals and electrolytes that make chicken broth so good for the soul. See page 191 for my Leftovers Chicken Stock recipe.

▶ **Up your enzymes.** Eat a spoonful of Homemade Sauerkraut (see page 200) or other fermented products with every meal. They produce a stack of helpful enzymes – which will assist the assimilation of the nutrition in the rest of your meal.

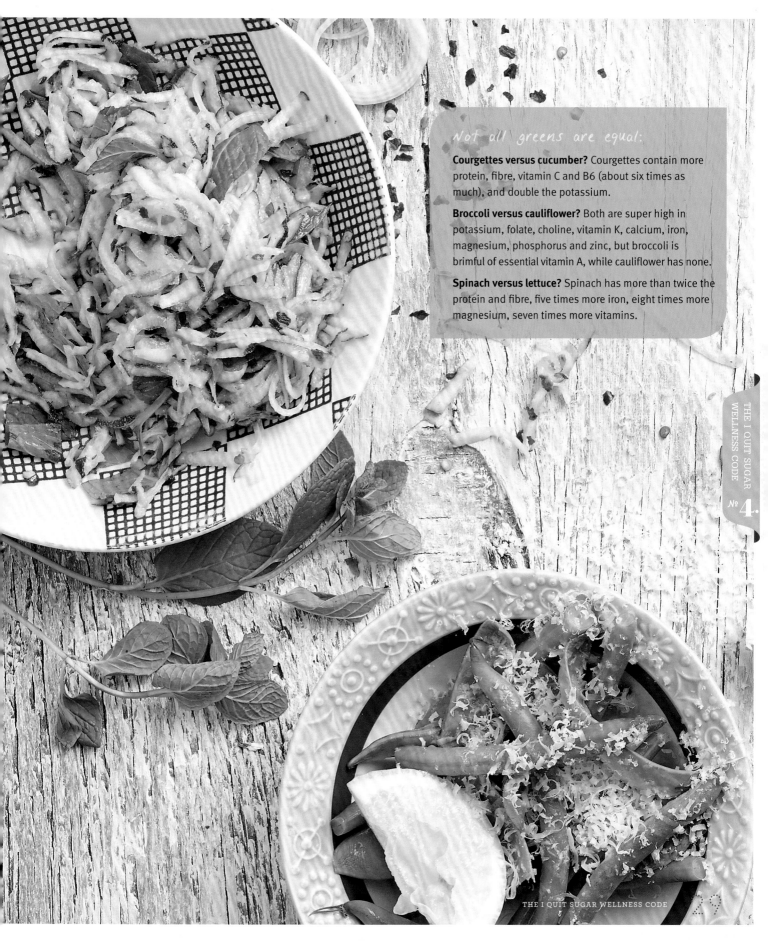

Not all greens are equal:

Courgettes versus cucumber? Courgettes contain more protein, fibre, vitamin C and B6 (about six times as much), and double the potassium.

Broccoli versus cauliflower? Both are super high in potassium, folate, choline, vitamin K, calcium, iron, magnesium, phosphorus and zinc, but broccoli is brimful of essential vitamin A, while cauliflower has none.

Spinach versus lettuce? Spinach has more than twice the protein and fibre, five times more iron, eight times more magnesium, seven times more vitamins.

LET'S TRY THIS

ADD MORE VEGETABLES TO YOUR LIFE

There are simple ways to do this, some of which are about 'disguising' (for kids and fussy eaters) their presence or replacing other less nutritious elements:

▶ **Add extra sides of greens. At every main meal** (see pages 128–9 for ideas).

▶ **Embed leafy greens.** Finely cut kale, spinach and Swiss chard, and add to soups, casseroles and pastas. They wilt down quickly and are easily disguised.

▶ **Smoothie green ice cubes.** Par-cook and purée (or leave whole) your greens (kale, broccoli, Swiss chard, pak choi, parsley), freeze in ice-cube trays and pop a few in your smoothie. Do up a bag of green ice cubes in bulk. (Note: par-cooking will reduce the goitrogenic effect of cruciferous vegetables like kale and broccoli.)

▶ **Sweeten sauces, soups and casseroles.** Add puréed pumpkin or sweet potato to red sauces (e.g. chilli dishes and curries) and 'yellow' cheesy dishes like mac 'n' cheese (see page 96).

▶ **Pack out your mashed potatoes and white sauces.** Add puréed cauliflower, turnip, swede or celeriac.

▶ **Replace some minced meat** with grated courgettes and carrot or finely cut mushrooms – easily disguised in tacos, bolognaise and meat loaf.

▶ **Flesh out just about anything.** Add broccoli, Swiss chard and cauliflower stalks – totally disguisable and a great way to use up these nutritious (and surprisingly sweet) bits.

▶ **Toss in some chia seeds.** Adding vegetables can up the liquid balance. Counter this with a teaspoon or two of chia seeds or chia bran.

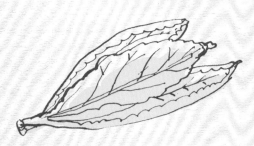

Q. WHAT BOOZE SHOULD I CHOOSE?

When you quit sugar, it doesn't mean you have to deny yourself. Responsible drinking is all good with caveats . . .

✔ Red wine: Contains minimal fructose. How so? It's the fructose in the grapes that ferments to become alcohol, leaving red wine low in sugar.

? White wine: Retains a little more of the fructose. Red is a better option.

? Champagne or 'sparkling': Tends to retain quite a lot of the sugar (fructose). Not a *great* option.

✔ Spirits: Dry spirits like gin, vodka and whisky are very low in fructose. But see the caveat on mixers below.

✔ Beer: Doesn't contain fructose. The sugar in beer and stout is maltose, which we can metabolise fine.

✘ Dessert wine: A stack of sugar remains unfermented. Don't touch the stuff.

? Apple cider: Retains quite a bit of fructose. Cloudy versions are the better option.

And a few words of advice . . .

⚠ Alcohol still has a multitude of metabolism and health issues that come with excessive consumption, not to mention it's addictive.

⚠ Only ever drink spirits with soda water or neat. Mixers, including tonic water, are full of sugar – about 8–10 teaspoons in one tall glass. Ditto fruit juices.

⚠ Me, I drink a glass of red wine with dinner 5–6 nights a week. I love an occasional dry gin martini, too. This works for me. I recommend no more than two drinks in any one sitting.

⚠ Always eat when you drink, to slow the rush of any sugar to the liver.

⚠ You may also find, once you cut out sugar, that your tolerance for alcohol is much lower.

⚠ Although alcohol is low in fructose it is still very high in empty calories. A beer is equivalent to a sausage roll. Two glasses of champagne is the equivalent of about one-fifth of your daily energy intake. Just sayin'!

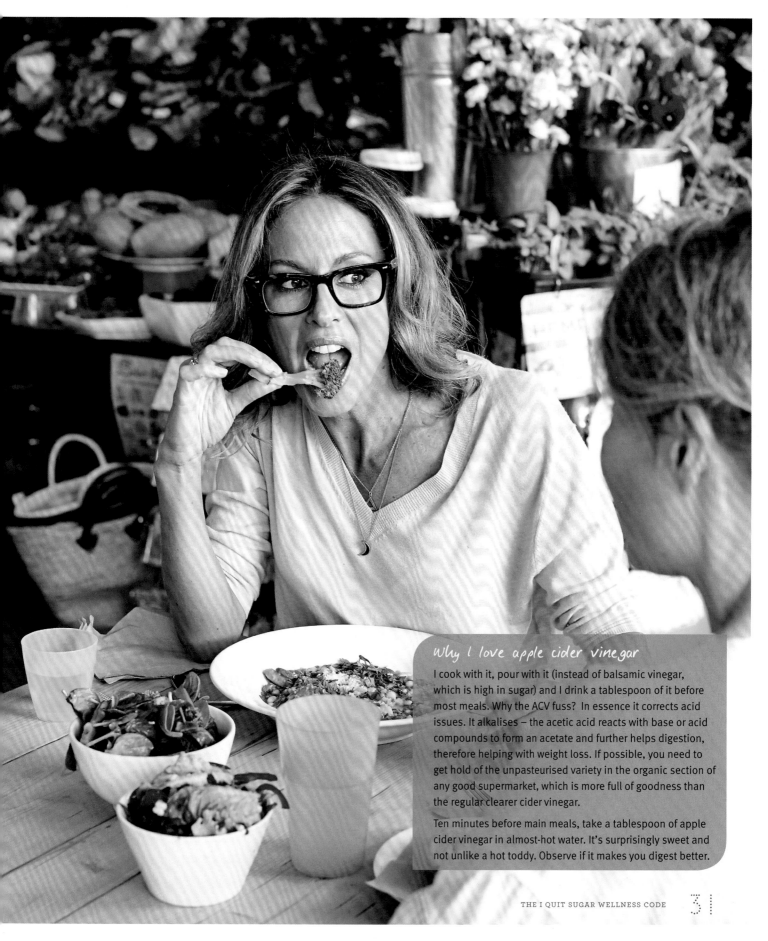

Why I love apple cider vinegar

I cook with it, pour with it (instead of balsamic vinegar, which is high in sugar) and I drink a tablespoon of it before most meals. Why the ACV fuss? In essence it corrects acid issues. It alkalises – the acetic acid reacts with base or acid compounds to form an acetate and further helps digestion, therefore helping with weight loss. If possible, you need to get hold of the unpasteurised variety in the organic section of any good supermarket, which is more full of goodness than the regular clearer cider vinegar.

Ten minutes before main meals, take a tablespoon of apple cider vinegar in almost-hot water. It's surprisingly sweet and not unlike a hot toddy. Observe if it makes you digest better.

How I EAT MORE GREENS

I'VE INVENTED A TERM: 'MISH-MASH MEALS'

They're simple breakfasts, lunches and dinners that moosh together a big stack of greenery with some protein, fat and highly satisfying 'cheat's flavourings'.

Here, I'll show you what I mean . . .

A clever way to add bonus 'cheat's flavouring': toss ⅓ cup (80 ml) of Homemade Sauerkraut (see page 200) through a mish-mash meal.

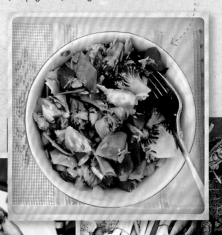

HOW TO USE UP LEFTOVER GREAT GRATED SALAD #1: mix with some peas, eggs, chopped bacon or ham and cheese and fry in an omelette pan.

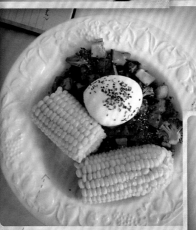

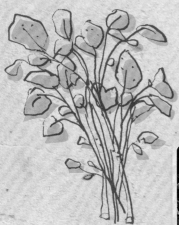

I start with Swiss chard and throw in tinned tuna, capers and olives. A handful of peas will lift a mish-mash meal.

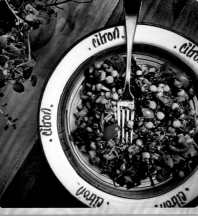

Q. DON'T CORN AND PEAS CONTAIN SUGAR?

Oh, look, sure they contain quite high amounts of sugar, but they're high in fibre, and I'm yet to meet anyone who binges on them or eats them by the bowlful. A handful in a meal for colour and kid-appeal is perfectly fine.

A poached or soft-boiled egg on top!

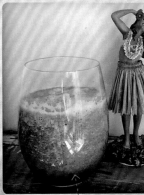

Any leftover greens go into my morning green smoothie.

One of my favourite 'cheat's flavourings': dulse flakes.

HOW TO USE UP LEFTOVER GREAT GRATED SALAD #2: When cooking up meatballs, sausage or mince, add leftover salad in the final stages of braising with a splash of apple cider vinegar and heat through. Oh, and some celery leaves, if they're hanging around.

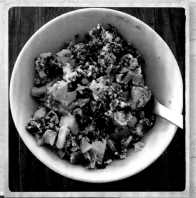

Par-Cooked 'n' Frozen Swiss chard and broccoli with 2 eggs and some grated cheddar 'scrambled' through it in a pan. This can also be done in the microwave at work. I tote the veggies straight from the freezer. Note: heat some avocado through your mish-mash – it adds lush creaminess.

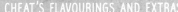

My Cheesy Green Mish-Mash Soup from my first book became a hit. I add 'cheat's flavouring' – 2 slices of grilled pancetta. Sometimes it's good to use meat just for a kick.

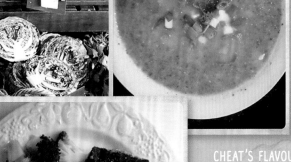

CHEAT'S FLAVOURINGS AND EXTRAS

Add these for extra salty and umami kick and all-in-one meal ease:

- Harissa paste
- Capers in salt (use the salt they come in instead of adding extra salt)
- Dulse flakes (instead of salt and for great iodine love)
- Homemade Sauerkraut (instead of vinegar and salt) (see page 200)
- Fermented Cucumbers
- Tinned tuna or sardines in extra-virgin olive oil (use the oil instead of adding extra oil; it's nice and flavoured with the fish)
- Olives (use the brine to braise or deglaze).

GREEN PIKELETS: Simply follow the instructions for Pumpkin Pikelets, but use Par-Cooked 'n' Frozen greens, puréed. I add a little feta and sometimes an egg and chia seeds to bind things better.

I start with some leftover sardines (see page 116) or tinned sardines and stir through parsley, rocket (or any other greenery, finely sliced), red onion and a little chilli (grate it straight from the freezer!). Plus olive oil and apple cider vinegar, or one of my dressings.

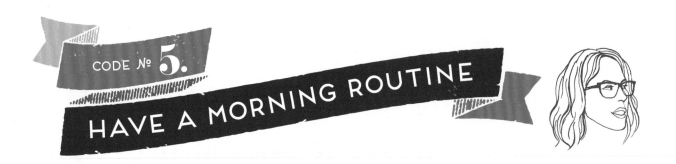

CODE № 5.

HAVE A MORNING ROUTINE

THE ONE THING EVERY INSPIRING THINKER I'VE INTERVIEWED (AND MANY BESIDES) SEEMS TO SHARE? A structured morning routine. A routine gets us moving, no brain required. It ejects us from stagnancy with purpose.

Benjamin Franklin always woke at 4 am and spent the morning reading and mapping out what he wanted to achieve that day. Obama does the same, always exercising before opening his first email no earlier than 9 am. Charles Darwin jumped straight from bed into exercise. P.G. Wodehouse always read a 'breakfast book'. For me, a morning routine sets the tone for the rest of my day – mindfulness and gentleness over frenetic toggling and reacting. It means I own my day, and am not dragged into it.

A GROUNDED START BEST SUPPORTS ME IN MY SUGAR-FREE WELLNESS.

I wake early and drink two to three glasses of warm water (boiled and left to cool a little) with a squeeze of lemon. Then I exercise (20–60 minutes). Then I meditate (20 minutes), shower and eat breakfast. It's taken years to set this habit in stone, but I do it without fail now, even when travelling.

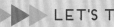

LET'S TRY THIS

CREATE A PERSONAL ROUTINE

First, set aside the time – it might be just 15 minutes. Get up a little earlier or sacrifice something (um, like checking your Instagram). Then choose whichever of the ideas below might get *you* sorted and set a good tone for *your* day. (Languid? Mindful? Focused?) It might take some experimenting. It did for me – probably a year or so before I settled into a groove that I looked forward to each day. Do your routine before breakfast (and before checking emails and feeds!):

1. Drink two to three glasses of warm water with a squeeze of lemon (the body absorbs warm water better; lemon juice alkalises the body, acts as a diuretic and activates the production of acids required for digestion, all of which serve to get your system moving).

2. Exercise. For ideas, see page 36. Morning is truly the best time to move, but I acknowledge it might not suit everyone.

3. Meditate or reflect quietly. Benjamin Franklin dedicated 5–7 am to the question, 'What good shall I do this day?' Getting gentle and grounded and certain provides the best launch pad for a productive day.

4. Read something inspiring or write. I'm always surprised how many leading thinkers do this religiously. Leo Barbauta from Zen Habits spent months paring his routine back to four things – drink water, sit on a cushion to reflect, read something inspiring, then start work. Julia Cameron's cultish book *The Artist's Way* advocates writing three 'morning pages' as soon as you wake, before doing anything else. This writing (a stream of consciousness of whatever comes to mind) unblocks your creativity and readies you for the day.

5. Write a list. Before plunging into emails, responding to what others want from you, work out *your* priorities.

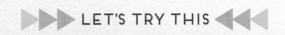

PACK A BETTER BREAKFAST

If you're reading this and using the line 'but a routine won't leave me time to eat my breakfast', give this a crack: take breakfast to work . . . in a jar. The breakfast packages below can be made the night before or in the morning while you're drinking your hot water with lemon – in a matter of minutes.

MONDAY	TUESDAY	WEDNESDAY	THURSDAY	FRIDAY

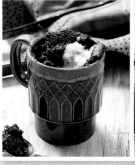 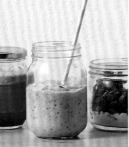 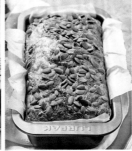 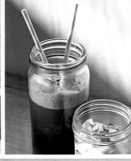 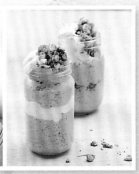

PALEO CHOC-COCO MUGGIN

Speed things up by pre-mixing the dry ingredients in bulk and dividing into zip-lock bags ready to dump into the mug with the liquid (see page 66).

3.5 minutes.

UP 'N' GO BREAKFAST WHIP

As much effort as whacking two Weetabix and some milk in a bowl, really (see page 84).

2.5 minutes.

PALEO INSIDE-OUT BREAD

Slice and freeze a loaf in batches of two. Stick in the toaster once you're in the office (see page 61).

1.5 minutes.

GREEN GLOWIN' SKIN SMOOTHIES

Have these with a handful of activated almonds. Speed things up: make double quantities – one for today, one for tomorrow (see pages 76–7).

2.5 minutes.

CARROT CAKE PORRIDGE WHIP

Make these the night before and just add your bits in the morning. Or, better, keep nuts and yoghurt at the office for adding on top once you're in there (see page 72).

30 seconds.

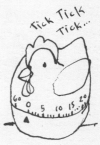

Tick Tick Tick...

THE I QUIT SUGAR WELLNESS CODE № 5.

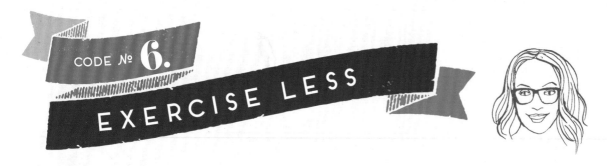

CODE № 6.

EXERCISE LESS

IT'S A CONTROVERSIAL IDEA, BUT HEAR ME OUT. Humans didn't evolve to blitz and pump and boot camp themselves silly in a gym and there's no evolutionary purpose to running marathons. Outrunning a sabre-toothed tiger for 2–3 hours was never going to be an accomplishable feat; we evolved to feed our energy to our brains so we could outsmart said tiger. In fact, we evolved to burn as little energy as possible during physical exertion.

To this end, exercise is a highly inefficient weight-loss technique. It's demotivating (it takes months to see a result), it sees us seek out more calories than we burn and we're programmed to return to our set-point, over and over (gosh, aren't genetics recalcitrant buggers!). To burn off one chocolate bar, you'd need to swim laps for more than an hour.

IQS MANTRA 6.

BACK THE FORK OFF Increasingly science (and my own experience . . . yours too?) is showing that going hard doesn't work. In fact, releasing our white-knuckled grip on life produces far better results. Of course, there are countless other health benefits to doing exercise. But the best results come from doing it mildly. Less is more, less is more . . .

What exercise is best?

30 minutes, *no more*, according to a Danish study, is optimal for fat loss, increasing aerobic capacity and reducing the risk of cardiovascular disease.

Shorter intervals are great too, found another study. Walking briskly for 10 minutes, three times a day, can be better than one long stint.

Mix it up. Other studies, however, show that mixing things up (shorter and longer workouts) is best. I, intuitively, agree.

Plus, the 'every day' bit is what counts. A 2012 study from the University of Wyoming found it takes three months of daily (moderate, casual) exercise before it starts to affect appetite control (for the better).

Forget weight loss . . . find another exercise raison d'être. Exercise for weight loss is not effective. Instead, think about using the promise of a clear head, fresh skin, agility and a vitamin D dose (instant results) as your motivator every day. Me, I view my morning workout as my grounding time. This is what gets me tying on my sneakers and out the door.

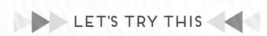

THE LESS-IS-MORE EXERCISE PLAN

Less stuff, less time, less fuss is the deal here. Try this approach for a month and see if it makes things smoother.

Exercise in the morning. It gets your circadian rhythms in synch and the greatest metabolic (and fat-burning) benefits are experienced at this time, and 'then it's done' – there's no risk of being too tired to do it later. You prefer afternoons? Cool, but I invite you to try mornings, just for a week as part of a morning routine and see how it fits.

Commit to 20 minutes only. This way you'll do it, you won't baulk (as you would if you bossily tell yourself you must do a 1-hour workout). Once started, you can bulk it up to 30 minutes if you're enjoying it. Or longer if it feels right for you.

Exercise every day. Something weird happens when you say you'll do it three days a week: you spend every morning deliberating whether *today* is one of those days instead of *just doing it*.

REMEMBER: FEWER DECISIONS MEAN MORE SELF-CONTROL MUSCLE FOR MORE IMPORTANT THINGS.

Exercise outside as often as possible. Studies show that our bodies respond better to the fresh air and connecting with nature. They call it the wilderness effect. Also, vitamin D from the sun assists our metabolism.

Exercise as close to home as possible. Don't waste time driving your bike to a park when you can ride straight from the front door. It's another complicating bit of palaver. Flow!

Keep fitness equipment absolutely minimal. And in one spot in the house, ready to go. No drink bottles, no fancy iPod carriers, no jangly keys (set aside one house key and put it in your shoe, pocket or down your bra). Equipment (looking for it, assembling it) can slow the momentum down and might even leave you with an excuse not to get it done.

TIE UP YOUR SHOELACES, GET OUT THE DOOR!

That said, buy a pedometer or download a walking app on your smartphone. This is a worthwhile investment. Counting your steps – and aiming for 10,000 a day – will get you competitive with yourself! I use the Moves app.

In addition: walk some more. For the rest of the day, find ways to walk more – to the supermarket, to meet friends for dinner, to get to work or university. Use Google Maps to work out the route and how long it will take. Or factor in the average pace of 5 kilometres per hour. Multitask (listen to podcasts or talking books or radio or return phone calls).

Do stair climbs. Got a park with steps nearby? Live in an apartment block or staying in a hotel? Do 20 minutes of laps, mixing up taking two steps at a time, jogging, etc. Alternatively, do laps up and down a steep hill.

Try a home workout on rainy days. There are heaps of short workout downloads on the Internet using everyday items such as tins of veggies, chairs, walls and your own body weight.

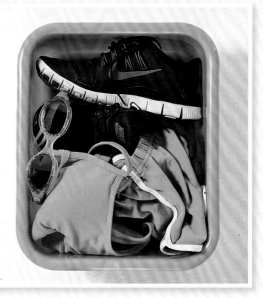

This is my exercise kit. I keep it in a pile in the laundry so I can grab it and 'literally' run. No hunting around for my sports bra.

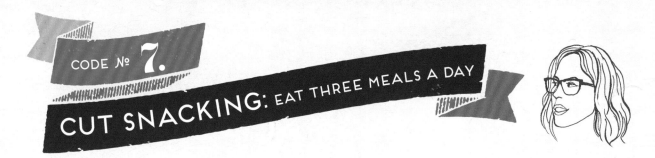

CODE № 7.

CUT SNACKING: EAT THREE MEALS A DAY

FACT: THE CONCEPT OF EATING 'SIX SMALL MEALS A DAY' AND SNACKING WAS DEVELOPED BY NUTRITIONISTS IN THE 1990s IN RESPONSE to everyone on the planet riding a blood-sugar roller-coaster and needing to fuel themselves every couple of hours.

The research that backed this approach pertained to diabetics. You could say it's a myth born as a paltry fix for sugar addiction. But most of us aren't designed to eat this way – it's inefficient and taxing on our bodies, which don't get the opportunity to rest between meals. An increasing number of studies are showing that bigger breaks between meals have big health benefits. Plus, there's this:

FULL MEALS TEND TO BE NUTRITIONALLY DENSE; SNACKS RARELY.

The good news: once you're off sugar for several months, you'll find you don't need to snack. Once again, it's about throwing a solid log (meals full of protein, with plenty of good fat) on the fire, instead of papery sugars. And getting on with the rest of our lives without the constant need to attend to our appetite.

 ## LET'S TRY THIS

CURBING THE SNACK ATTACKS

Most of the time when I think I'm hungry between meals it's more a case of my not being *quite* satiated . . . *yet*. In such cases I find it helpful to:

▶ **Wait 15–20 minutes.** Sometimes my metabolism is slow to react. Wait a little – go for a walk, run an errand – and then see if you're still hungry.

▶ **Drink some water.** Quite often hunger is actually thirst.

▶ **Eat a tablespoon of coconut oil** (see page 16). This works 100% and for a good few hours. Promise!

▶ **If I'm genuinely hungry between meals, I eat.** I recommend nuts, cheese or yoghurt. They can be found most places (even in service stations) and they work fast.

 ## LET'S TRY THIS

EATING FULL MEALS

I believe most people do not eat enough – at least enough dense nutrition – and particularly at lunch. I was the same for years. I'd get all modest with my midday meal, then turn to snacks (sweet ones) around 3 pm. It took several visits to Europe to get a good feel for how a meal should be eaten. Over there, women and men alike commit to a proper lunch that fills them up until dinner. They don't do afternoon tea and snacks are not de rigueur. Some things to try:

▶ Eat a handful-sized serve of protein at breakfast, lunch and dinner.

▶ Include at least 2 cups of vegetables at lunch and dinner. If it's a salad, it should be 3 cups.

▶ While adjusting to this 'three meals only' way of eating, add an extra boiled egg (or two) or feta cheese (a proper slab) to your meal if you get hungry. Throw on some seeds, nuts and, of course, a good glug of oil or dressing like the Europeans do.

▶ Don't be shy about including several elements. I'll often eat a soup or broth *and* a box of leftover roast vegetables *and* a leftover chop.

Cinnamon and all things nice

Why do I add cinnamon to my 'sweet' recipes? Along with turmeric, cloves and bay leaves, it stimulates insulin activity (indeed, triples it) and helps process sugar more efficiently.

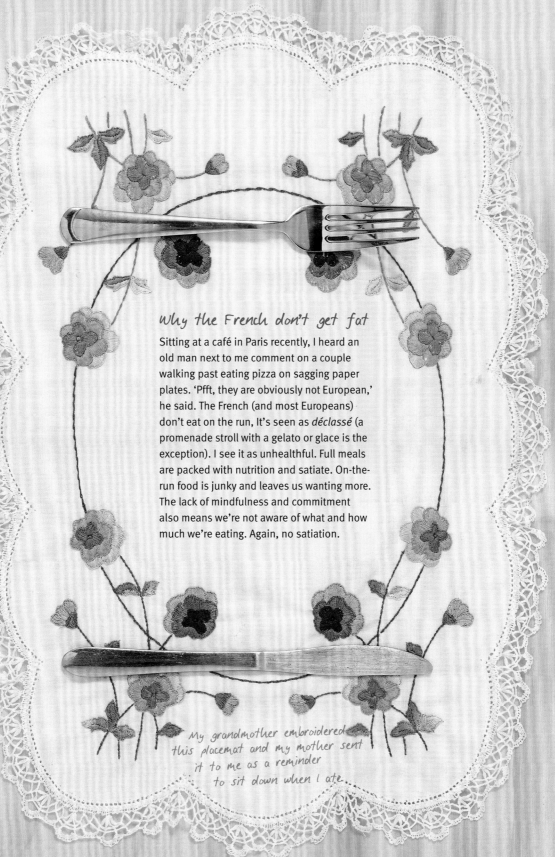

Why the French don't get fat

Sitting at a café in Paris recently, I heard an old man next to me comment on a couple walking past eating pizza on sagging paper plates. 'Pfft, they are obviously not European,' he said. The French (and most Europeans) don't eat on the run, It's seen as *déclassé* (a promenade stroll with a gelato or glace is the exception). I see it as unhealthful. Full meals are packed with nutrition and satiate. On-the-run food is junky and leaves us wanting more. The lack of mindfulness and commitment also means we're not aware of what and how much we're eating. Again, no satiation.

My grandmother embroidered this placemat and my mother sent it to me as a reminder to sit down when I ate.

I GET ASKED THIS QUESTION MORE THAN ANY – HOW DO I NAVIGATE WELLNESS WHEN I'M NOT IN MY USUAL ROUTINE?

It can be tricky, but I have my ways.

Yes, they're a little unconventional, but it's become part of my flow.

HIKE. *It's a wonderful raison d'être for travelling.*

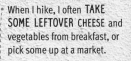

When I hike, I often TAKE SOME LEFTOVER CHEESE and vegetables from breakfast, or pick some up at a market.

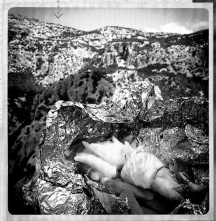

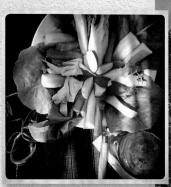

A nutrient-dense fix: CRUDITÉS.

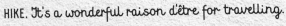

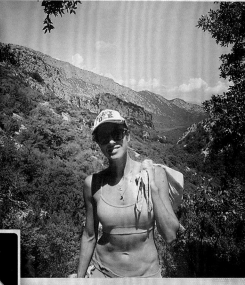

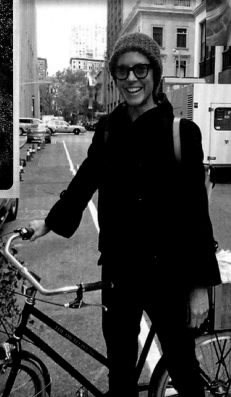

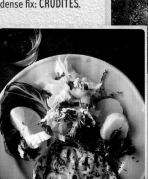

EAT AS THE LOCALS DO.
What they're choosing will often be in season and high quality.

SALAD BARS in big cities can be a pretty good option. Go for oven-roasted or steamed vegetables, roast meats or steamed fish. But avoid the 'salads', they're usually drenched in dressing (ergo drenched in sugar).

USE CITY BIKE SCHEMES. Many major cities have them now. They are cheap and the best way to get around a city.

EMBRACE TOTALLY TOTE-ABLES (see page 71) for road trips and on short-haul plane rides. I pack a green smoothie wherever I go, then use the canister as a water bottle for the rest of the trip.

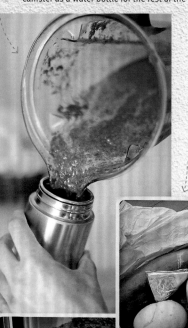

Another SIMPLE HIKING LUNCH pulled from the markets and the breakfast buffet at the hotel/hostel.

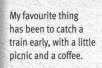

My favourite thing has been to catch a train early, with a little picnic and a coffee.

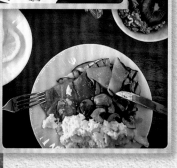

AT BREAKFAST BUFFETS I GO FOR EGGS, any vegetable matter I can find, low-fructose fruit and extra, clean protein.

▶ GET DENSE AT RESTAURANTS AND CAFÉS by seeking out bowls of greens at every opportunity. I always look to the 'sides' section of a menu – if they do a steamed seasonal greens dish, I'm sorted. I only need to focus on good protein from there.

▶ CHOOSE THE LEAST INGREDIENTS. Favour the steak, roast chicken, slow-cooked lamb, grilled or baked fish over pastas, pizzas, stir-fries and any other dishes that involve goobie sauces and things that can't be immediately identified.

▶ AVOID CARBS. I tend to do this when I travel. In part because convenience carbs (the ones you're most likely to eat on the move) are often processed, sugary and gluten (toxin) heavy. Also because they generally come covered in sugar-laden sauces (to balance the stodge factor). And finally because they're cheap calories.

▶ PACK GREEN POWDERS to ensure you're getting enough vitamins and minerals. Many come in individual serve sachets that you can pour into a bought smoothie or even just into water at breakfast or lunch. I also pack protein powders, again the ones that come in individual sachets.

▶ PACK BREAKFAST BAGS. I mix up some linseeds, nuts, chia seeds and coconut shreds in zip-locks ready to dump into yoghurt or milk on planes, in meetings or in hotels.

▶ LOAD UP AT BREAKFAST, especially at hotels or hostels where breakfast is included. This means lunch can be a lesser deal.

▶ HAVE A NUTRITION-DENSE FIX A DAY. I swap a meal (lunch is best) for a really simple 'snack' of raw beans, a cucumber, a head of chicory, a chunk of cheese – whatever I can find at a market or deli.

▶ ON THE ROAD. At service stations and late night convenience stores you can grab plain yoghurt, nuts, a little block of cheddar cheese and a packet of rice cakes.

▶ EXERCISE DAILY, AS A PRIORITY. To clear your lymphs and get everything moving right (travel constipates, disrupts Vata and slows everything down). Doing weights at a hotel gym is great when travelling – they don't sap energy as much as cardio and get the joints moving. If there's no gym, I run the fire stairs in the hotel.

▶ STEAM. Make use of a hotel sauna/steam room. Steam is so good for clearing your lymph glands and getting gunk out of your system.

▶ WALK. It's the best way to see a city, often faster and ticks off exercise.

▶ ON PLANES. I wear pressure socks to ensure my lymphs don't get blocked up. Also, drink loads of water and meditate to bring your Vata energy down.

▶ I PACK LAVENDER OIL – for better sleep and to put on pimples (which I always get when travelling).

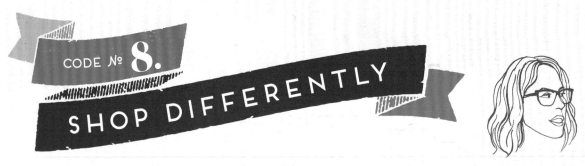

CODE № **8.**

SHOP DIFFERENTLY

I'M OFTEN ASKED HOW I SHOP – ORGANIC? FREE-RANGE? ETHICAL? SEASONAL? ACCORDING TO THE LEAST FOOD MILES? As a rule, I prioritise the environment and ethics over my personal health, and work to two principles...

1. I shop as local as possible.

Why? It's a good catch-all approach. I buy as much as I can from local markets where the farmers sell direct. Elsewhere I always check the label to see that it hasn't travelled around the world to get to the shelf. This ticks off the *food miles* and *seasonality* concern. It also often ticks off the *ethical* and *organic* issues. Local farmers are more likely to connect with the community and its ecological concerns.

2. I don't waste.

I use up my scraps, reinvent my leftovers and store things properly so they don't go off. This contributes more to the planet – and my hip pocket – than any other approach. The biggest environmental issue on the planet, contributing more to carbon emissions than cars and industry? Food wastage. The biggest factor in the food wastage chain? Us (not the farmers or the supermarkets). The biggest hit to our hip pocket when food shopping? Tossing out food we don't use.

By focusing on these two things only, you might find you can shop with clarity and conscience, too.

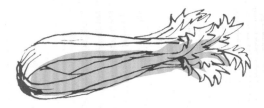

HOW TO SHOP WELL

Where possible it is better to buy organic, for a host of important reasons. But for many, organic fare just ain't affordable. Here's how you can prioritise your spending if you care about chemicals in your dinner. (One caveat: I personally do not endorse buying, for example, celery from California, just because it's organic. Local trumps this kind of craziness.)

CHICKEN AND EGGS – ALWAYS BUY ORGANIC

Free-range birds might be able to move outside a cage but they can still be fed nasty chemical-laden feed and supplements. Many authorities, including CHOICE, say it's worth investing in organic chook products. Bear in mind, with IQS we cook the whole chook, often slowly, to extract as much nutrition as possible. We certainly don't want to be leaching residual chemicals into our soup too! But keep it affordable . . .

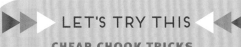

▶▶▶ LET'S TRY THIS ◀◀◀

CHEAP CHOOK TRICKS

▶ **Eat the unfashionable bits.** Drumsticks and wings are often a fraction of the cost of the more fashionable breast.

▶ **Eat the whole bird.** A whole chook works out to be very economical. Especially if you . . .

▶ **Extend it further.** I can make a $20 organic chook stretch to 15 meals.

▶ **Make stock.** This means you use every last bit of the bird.

BEEF AND LAMB –
ORGANIC AND PASTURE-FED IS BEST

Increasingly, an important consideration when shopping for red meat is: is it pasture- or grain-fed? The latter can present a host of ethical, health and environmental issues (the animals are kept in small lots, the grains up the omega-6 count of the meat, and using fertile land for animal grain is wasteful).

Having said that, in Australia, unlike most of the world, most lamb and 70% of beef is pasture-fed and raised on arid rangelands where nothing else can be grown (no fertile land is wasted). Hoorah! Cattle tends to be grain-fed only in times of drought and even then just 'grain-finished'. Only occasionally is meat specifically grown to be grain-fed, so it's easy to avoid.

So, the main issue here is the organic factor. Non-organic beef can be treated with growth-promoting hormones. It might say a lot to you that the European Union has banned growth hormones and deemed them a health risk, and that Australia deems them unfit for chooks but not red meat.

 LET'S TRY THIS ◀◀

CHEAP RED MEAT TRICKS

▶ **Buy tough, unfashionable cuts.** Cuts such as chuck, brisket, shin, osso bucco and shanks are much cheaper than sirloins.

▶ **Slow-cook your meat.** Which, in turn, means you use less meat (since you bulk it out with vegetables) but get maximum flavour, and extra nutritional bang from extracting minerals and gelatine from the meat, while preserving enzymes (see page 28).

FRUIT AND VEGGIES –
ORGANIC (SOMETIMES)

There are three types of produce that tend to retain chemical residues and thus it is best to buy organic:

1. Soft-fleshed fruit, such as stone fruit and berries.

2. Veggies where you eat the skin, such as carrots, broccoli, peppers and celery.

3. Leafy greens, such as lettuce and spinach, and leafy herbs such as parsley and coriander.

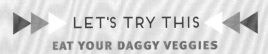 LET'S TRY THIS ◀◀

EAT YOUR DAGGY VEGGIES

The daggier the veg, the cheaper it is. I almost treat it as a sport – buying up the veg no one else eats (or has heard of) and finding fresh ways to use them. This simple game is a great way to vary your diet and support seasonality. Look out for these in the supermarket:

Swede: With a yellow and purplish skin, this relative of the turnip can be found in most supermarkets with the root veg. Steam and mash as you would parsnip or turnip, dice and add to soups or cut into batons and eat raw (as I do – it's super-sweet!).

Chicory: When in season, this torpedo-shaped sweet-bitter clump of white-yellow leaves often comes in economical packs of three or four. Slice into salads, pull apart the cupped leaves and use as you would a wrap or taco or dipping chip, or just eat raw (it's a great hiking food as it is densely packed). You can also braise it to bring out its sweetness.

Marrow: These are a large vegetable that are super cheap in summer. They have a mild flavour and don't need to be peeled. Stuff them, bake them, steam and serve with plenty of butter.

FISH –
ALWAYS BUY SUSTAINABLE

There are a bunch of complicated considerations for buying the best kind of fish. A good idea is to download an app listing sustainable fish. In Australia, the Australian Marine Conservation Society (AMCS) is the authority and their Sustainable Seafood Guide app is great. However, here are some general rules de thumb (which are also economical):

▶ **Go for white-fleshed** (pollack, mahi mahi, mullet, whiting or coley).

▶ **Avoid big predators,** such as southern bluefin tuna, shark (flake), striped marlin and swordfish, in part because they're chronically overfished and reproduce slowly, but also because, being at the top of the food chain, they contain large amounts of mercury.

▶ **If you do eat tuna** go for skipjack tuna rather than southern bluefin, yellowfin or bigeye, which are overfished.

▶ **Go for small** and fast-growing fish, which can replenish more quickly if their stocks are affected.

▶ **Avoid farmed salmon.** Farms use antibiotics and that causes environmental issues, and the salmon are fed using large quantities of smaller fish we'd be better off eating directly. Go for wild-caught salmon instead.

CHEAP FISH TRICKS

Try sardines. Have you ever bought them fresh? Seriously, they're dirt cheap, stupidly good for you and one of the most sustainable options at the fishmonger. I cook them on a sheet of foil under the grill and eat on toast with some homemade mayo and mustard. I smash grilled fresh sardines or tinned ones with lemon, pepper, chilli flakes and parsley and spread on top of avocado toast.

Look out for fish offcuts. These are often less than half the price of the full thing and can be used to make soup, stews or nugget-style fish 'n' chips. When I want to eat salmon, I buy salmon tails which have lots of lovely skin on them (the most nutritious bit of the fish, so please don't discard it!).

 Q. WHAT TINNED TUNA IS BEST?

Most canned tuna is caught using FADS, destructive and unethical nets and trawling equipment. Always opt for pole and line varieties – this style of fishing is more selective, meaning it can avoid unsustainable species, such as bigeye and yellowfin. Most of the big tinned tuna brands are gradually swapping to this approach. It will say 'pole and line' on the can and you'll find they're the same price as regular tuna. I've supported this cause for a few years and you can find more on my blog, sarahwilson.com.au.

LET'S TRY THIS

BUY OUT-OF-DATE

Much food wastage occurs because we think food is old and unsafe to eat. But the 'use-by date' and 'best before date' are different things. The former tells you when a food must be eaten for health and safety reasons. The best before date gives an indication of when it's best to eat. But supermarkets can still sell it after that date.

So, if meat or fish is marked down because the best before date is approaching, buy it up and freeze it. I do. The quality will be preserved instantly. Just ensure that you consume it within two to three months and that you don't refreeze it once thawed.

RECIPE TO TRY

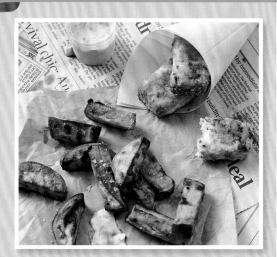

SUSTAINABLE FISH 'N' CHIPS (see page 90)
This recipe uses white-fleshed offcuts.

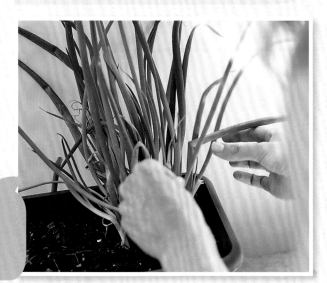

SUSTAINABLE TIP: When I buy a bunch of spring onions, I immediately plonk it in a pot of soil. It will stay 'alive' for weeks, even months.

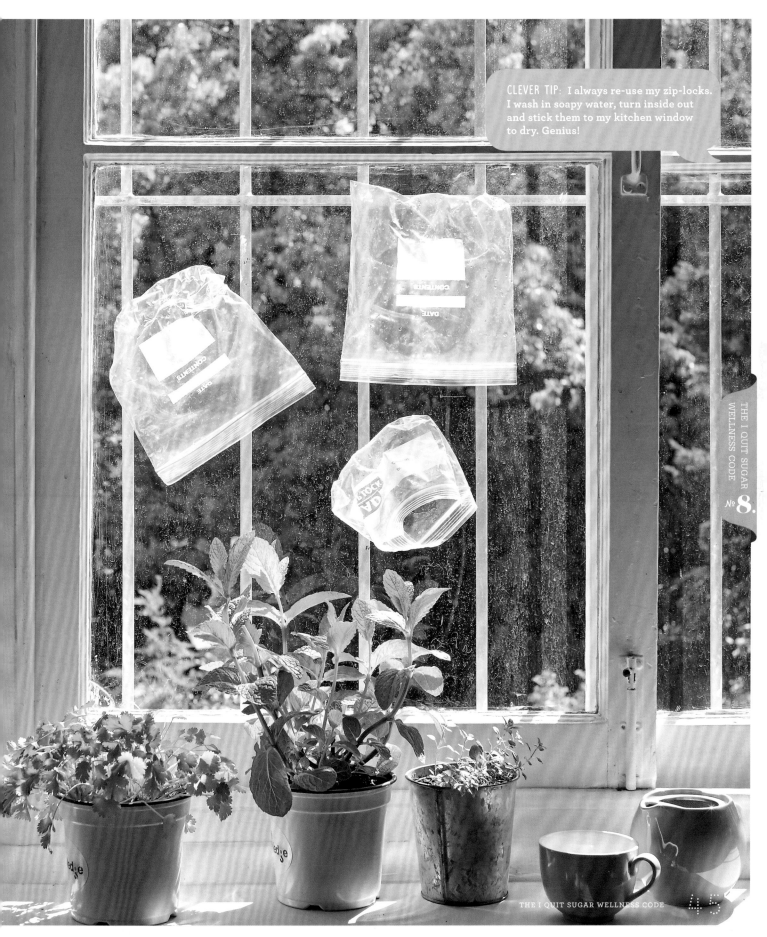

CLEVER TIP: I always re-use my zip-locks. I wash in soapy water, turn inside out and stick them to my kitchen window to dry. Genius!

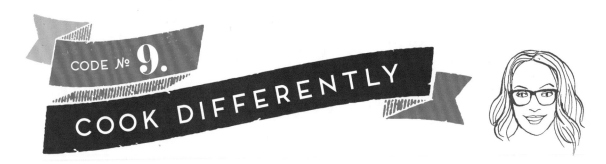

CODE № 9.
COOK DIFFERENTLY

THIS FINAL CODE IS A CULMINATION OF MOST OF THE STUFF THAT'S COME BEFORE IT. Cooking empowers us to live how we want to live, unencumbered by addiction and low-brow choices. It enables wellness. Author and food activist Michael Pollan says, 'Not cooking breeds helplessness, dependence and ignorance.'

The way we cook can empower us even further. These simple techniques, which we'll be using throughout the recipe section of this book, ensure we waste less and maximise dense nutrition. They allow us to live well with less restriction and more flow. And without sugar.

IQS MANTRA 7.

FLOW Find ways and means to cut the palaver, the fuss, the fitness equipment, the recipe steps and ingredients, the cooking vessels, your possessions, your hesitancy and live more smoothly. We need to feel free. Full wellness is about feeling free and flowy.

This means learning how to cook in simpler, smarter and more down-to-earth, no-brainer ways. Like our grandmothers used to. Too often recipes demand we head out to buy new ingredients and use 92,347 dishes and steps. They pay no heed to what happens to leftovers and scraps, nor do they show us how to flow what we've cooked into extra meals, or how to bulk-cook so we don't have to go through the very same ordeal next time we cook.

We can learn this ourselves, though.

GET EQUIPPED

There's often no need to go out and buy special equipment. Work with what you've got. That said, if you do wish to invest in a few bits of equipment, I recommend the following:

▶ **An electric slow cooker** These things are super-cheap. It doesn't have to be a big one (mine is a 4.5-litre model, and easily makes 6–8 portions). Make sure you get one with a timer though. Sadly, I didn't!

▶ **A stick blender or 'stab-mixer'** These are sold individually or as part of a blender ensemble.

▶ **A high-powered blender** Expensive, but key to making green smoothies. I use mine every day.

▶ **BPA-free freezer containers** I explain further over on page 50.

LEARN TO SLOW-COOK

Why? Because it ticks off so many Wellness Code boxes. Slow-cooking preserves enzymes in meat and vegetables because we cook at low temperatures and it extracts the cartilage, marrow and minerals (denser nutrition!). It demands the use of economical cuts of meat that can be otherwise discarded – shanks, neck, shins, cheeks and chuck – as these are the best cuts to slow-cook. Plus, because this 'slow 'n' low' approach extracts so much flavour from any meat used, you can use less of it, 'fleshing' things out with cheap veggies and starches.

Why an electric slow cooker? First, it's the ultimate one-step, one-pot wonder. You just chuck everything in and press a button. Second, it uses about the same amount of electricity as a light bulb and about one-third the CO_2 of an oven. And, since you leave it on during the day, it's using power from the grid at a low-demand time.

If you don't have a slow cooker, you can use a heavy-based casserole pot instead. Or a cast-iron casserole on the stovetop or in the oven. You'll need to add extra liquid (about double) if you do, and reduce the cooking time from 8 hours (on low) or 4 hours (on high) to 1–2 hours.

CUT STAGES AND POTS
The recipes in this book are designed to be one-pot wonders with three steps or less in as many cases as possible. I actively encourage you to cheat further:

▶ **Use your blender as a mixing bowl.** Do any grating, whipping or puréeing first, then add the remaining ingredients directly into the blender to stir with a spoon or lightly blend.

▶ **Cook pasta and rice in your sauce** to save pots. I realise this is hardly elegant, but for midweek meals, why not? A 1:1 pasta-to-sauce ratio is best (1:2 rice-to-sauce). Add more if your sauce is particularly chunky. Cook for the same time as you would normally.

▶ **Use an overproof pan.** Sometimes dishes require sautéing on the stovetop *then* placing in a new dish *then* placing under a grill or in the oven for browning. Streamline things by cooking in an ovenproof pan or casserole dish and transferring the one dish around the kitchen.

▶ **Use a double steamer.** Or a steaming colander over a saucepan, and boil your starchy vegetables, or even your casserole or soup, on the bottom while steaming your greens up top. Just watch it doesn't boil over.

USE YOUR LEFTOVERS
The average Australian tosses out 20% of their weekly shop. The waste kills me. The claim that many of us can't afford good food also kills me when the painfully obvious thing to do is to cut costs by cutting waste. Catch my simple drift? For leftover ideas, flick to Brilliant Leftovers, page 187.

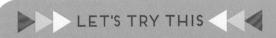

▶▶▶ LET'S TRY THIS ◀◀◀
COOKING WITH A SLOW COOKER

A few things to bear in mind:

▶ **Cook in bulk.** Slow cookers work best when filled to two-thirds of capacity. If that's more than you need, freeze the leftovers.

▶ **The order matters.** Put your densest veggies on the bottom. Place your meat on top of the veggies. Sauces over the top of that. Soft veg, like courgettes and peas, should be added in the last 30 minutes. Ditto dairy and seafood.

▶ **Don't check on the pot once it's started cooking.** You'll only extend the cooking time if you lift the lid and let moisture and heat escape. If you have to open it (to add ingredients), whack it on high for 20 minutes.

▶ **And if the final product is too runny,** just add a tablespoon or two of arrowroot, cornflour or chia seeds to thicken it out. Or reserve some of the juices and use as a lovely, rich stock in other dishes.

▶ **Skip the pre-brown step when slow-cooking.** It does add extra caramelisation, but I find enough flavour is drawn from the slow-cooking itself.

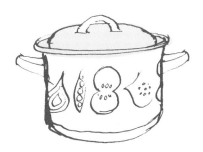

How to use your FREEZER better

HONESTLY, MY GO-TO ADVICE WHEN ANYONE ASKS ME TO
SHARE THE SMARTEST THING I DO: BULK-BUY 'N' FREEZE.

I buy up when a product is in season (when it's cheap and
abundant), prepare it in bulk (saving time) and then freeze it ready
to use later. Besides the obvious environmental and economic
savings, there's this:

A FULL FREEZER IS MORE ENERGY EFFICIENT THAN AN EMPTY ONE.

Why? Because solids freeze at
a lower temperature than air,
requiring less electricity.

▶▶▶ LET'S TRY THIS ◀◀◀

FRIDGE SURPRISE

Open your fridge and see what's in there. Create a
meal around what you find. The ultimate challenge:
not to buy anything extra. Use substitutes if you have
to. Draw on your freezer stash. If you happen to love
the result, feel free to share it with me on instagram
(@_sarahwilson_) with the hashtag #fridgesurprise.

Use cookbooks or recipe apps that list things based on
the ingredient (I love Stephanie Alexander's *The Cook's
Companion* for this). If you have two aubergines, look
up recipes that are aubergine-based.

BULK-BUY 'N' FREEZE

Buy up the following in large amounts when they're in season:

▶ **Avocados.** Purée with coconut water and/or coconut cream and a little lime juice. Freeze in ice-lolly moulds to eat as lollies or to pop out and blend with some extra greens to make a nutritious smoothie. Feel free to replace the lime with raw cacao for a choc version.

▶ **Lemons and limes.** Juice and freeze in ice-cube trays ready for smoothies.

▶ **Onions, celery, peppers, tomatoes.** Dice and freeze ready for soups and casseroles.

▶ **Courgettes.** Dice and freeze, as above, or grate and freeze in ice-cube trays ready to pop out and use to 'dense out' meat dishes, omelettes or soup.

▶ **Kale, Swiss chard, broccoli.** Par-Cook 'n' Freeze as per page 51. You can also purée them and freeze in ice-cube trays ready to pop into smoothies.

▶ **Cauliflower.** Par-Cook 'n' Freeze or grate raw (to make cauliflower 'rice') and freeze ready to make Cauliflower 'Fried Rice' (page 100) or my cauliflower pizza base (page 98).

▶ **Beetroot.** Par-Cook 'n' Freeze as per page 51.

▶ **Pumpkin and sweet potato.** Again Par-Cook 'n' Freeze, purée (as per page 51) ready to bulk out meals and to make Sweet Potato Casserole (page 111) and Snickery Pumpkin Mud Smoothie (page 74).

▶ **Mince.** Make a batch of mince into meatballs or patties and freeze, uncooked, ready to make my Deconstructed Hamburger (see page 88).

▶ **Egg Whites.** Freeze each white in an ice-cube tray. Then transfer to a freezer container. Make sure you thaw them completely before using – they'll beat better at room temperature.

▶ **Egg Yolks.** Gelation causes the yolks to thicken, becoming too gluggy to use when frozen, so whisk ⅛ teaspoon salt or 1½ teaspoons rice malt syrup per 4 yolks.

▶ **Bacon.** It can be a chore to fry up if you're only using it for flavouring (as I often do). Dice and cook a pack in one go, ready to crumble on top of soups or add to eggs.

▶ **Fresh herbs.** See page 194.

▶ **Whole berries.** Place in the freezer ready for smoothies (no need to use ice).

▶ **Nuts and seeds.** Store in the freezer. They keep fresher this way and won't go rancid. Better still, activate them and then freeze.

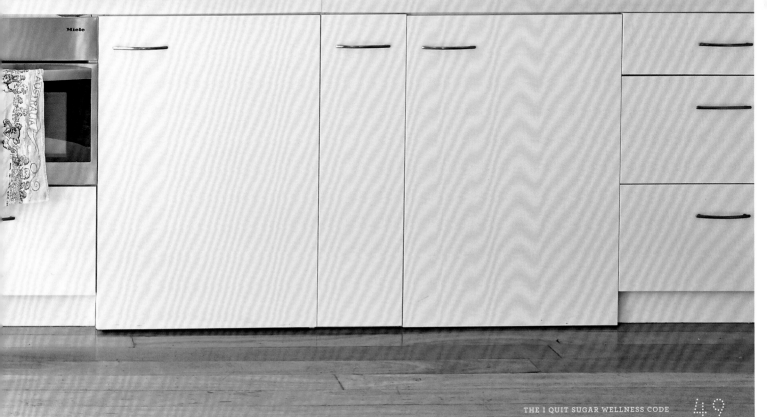

KNOW HOW LONG TO FREEZE YOUR FOOD

As far as food safety is concerned, freezing food for any length of time is safe. However, flavour and visuals can be compromised.

▶ **Meat soups:** 2 months.

▶ **Vegetable soups:** 3 months.

▶ **Par-Cooked 'n' Frozen vegetables:** 3–6 months. Generally they don't need to be defrosted prior to cooking, although some leafy green vegetables are much easier to separate if defrosted a little bit first.

▶ **Cooked meat:** 2 months. If possible, slightly undercook any meat that is going to be reheated.

▶ **Cooked fish:** 1 month.

▶ **Baked muffins:** 3 months. Freeze in individual bags or in a single container with sheets of freezer paper between the muffins so they can be easily separated.

FINESSING YOUR FREEZING SKILLS

▶ Label your foods as they go into the freezer with the date by which they should be used.

▶ Defrost foods in the fridge, not on the worktop. The slower you defrost, the closer it resembles its pre-frozen state.

▶ Wrappin' good: glass and ceramic containers, brown paper bags or paper (not greaseproof) are your best options, but not always practical. The good news: cling film is now much safer (no longer made from PVC) and there are safer BPA-free plastic lunchboxes now.

▶ Freeze things in a thin layer in your zip-lock bag, so you can 'snap' off what you need as you go.

▶ When freezing things in ice-cube trays, transfer your frozen cubes to a zip-lock bag, to free up your tray.

▶ Keep a large zip-lock bag in the freezer, and pop in your cooking scraps of chicken, meat bones, fish bones and heads, and vegetable trimmings (keep separate bags for different meats). When it's full, make a stock (see my Leftovers Chicken Stock recipe on page 191).

HOW TO COOK WITH MY RECIPES

CHOOSE OUR OWN (DIETARY) ADVENTURE

You'll notice each recipe comes with a bunch of little coloured icons denoting dietary needs. In some cases the meal will be easily adaptable to the particular dietary need. The icons mean:

 PALEO/GLUTEN-FREE

 VEGAN/DAIRY-FREE

 SUPERGREEN
(for the Cleanse Week recipes)

 8WP (for things to eat when going through quitting process i.e. non-sweet things)

SOLO COOKERS: any recipes serving 4 can be eaten over several days (I provide tips along the way) or extra portions can be frozen

FOURSOME FAMILY: simply quadruple relevant recipes

There are a number of staples I suggest you have in your freezer at all times. Start with these.

PUMPKIN PURÉE

Preheat the oven to 180°C (gas 4). Scoop out and discard the pumpkin seeds and pulp. Put the pumpkin wedges on a baking tray, then rub with the olive oil and salt. Bake on the middle oven rack until tender – about 1 hour. (If you're pressed for time, cut the pumpkin into smaller chunks and bake for 30 minutes.) Scoop out the flesh and purée using a stick blender or mash well by hand. Once cool, store in 1-cup (250 ml) batches in the freezer in zip-lock bags or sealed containers. You can also use this recipe to make sweet potato purée (approximately 4 sweet potatoes to 1 large pumpkin).

1 large pumpkin, cut into 4 big wedges
2 tablespoons olive oil
pinch of salt

PAR-COOKED 'N' FROZEN VEGGIES

▶ **Buy a stash of veggies.** Stock up on your favourite vegetables when they are in season or on special. Organic veggies can often be really cheap at certain times of the year – invest when they are. Mix it up. Broccoli, spinach, beetroot, kale, beans and cauliflower work really well as a mixture, but you can try other veggies too.

▶ **Using a saucepan with a steamer** (or double steamer), steam the veggies for 1–2 minutes, then rinse in cold water to stop the cooking process. For beetroots, place them on a tray (no oil or salt) and bake at 180°C (gas 4) for 20–30 minutes until tender.

▶ **Drain and freeze in portions.** I divide mine into per-serve portions and put them in zip-lock bags. You can also dump them all into one large container and 'break off' what you need as you go, as you would frozen peas.

SOME OTHERS TO STOCK UP ON . . .

✳ Activated Nuts (see page 204)

✳ Whey (see page 204)

✳ Bone Broth (see page 190)

✳ Leftovers Chicken Stock (see page 191)

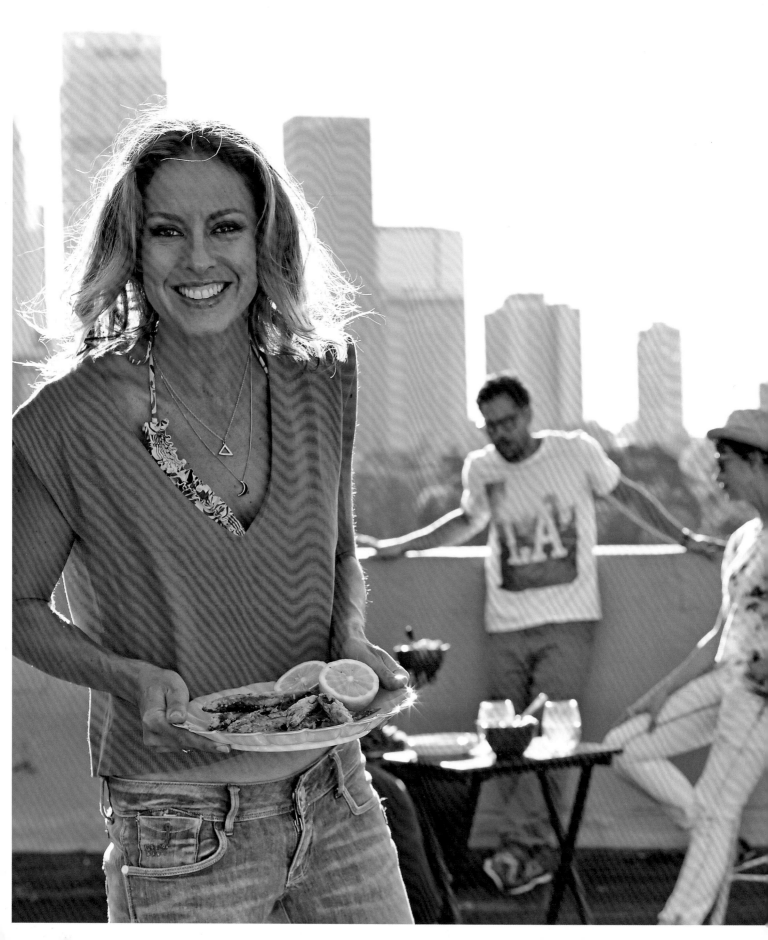

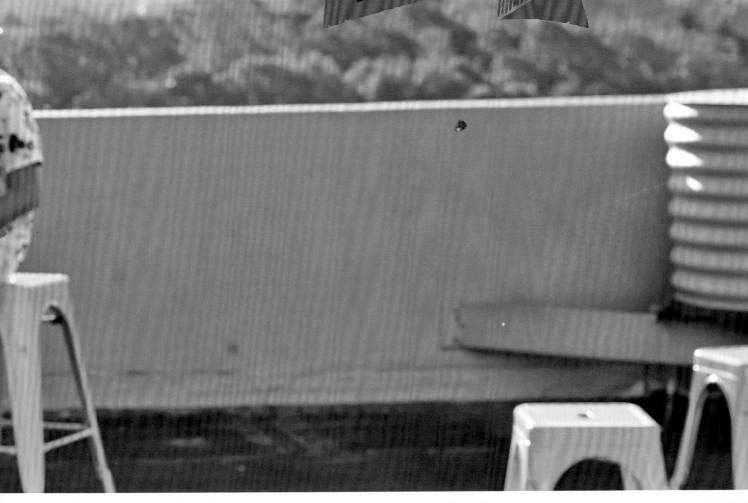

148
SUGAR-FREE
RECIPES

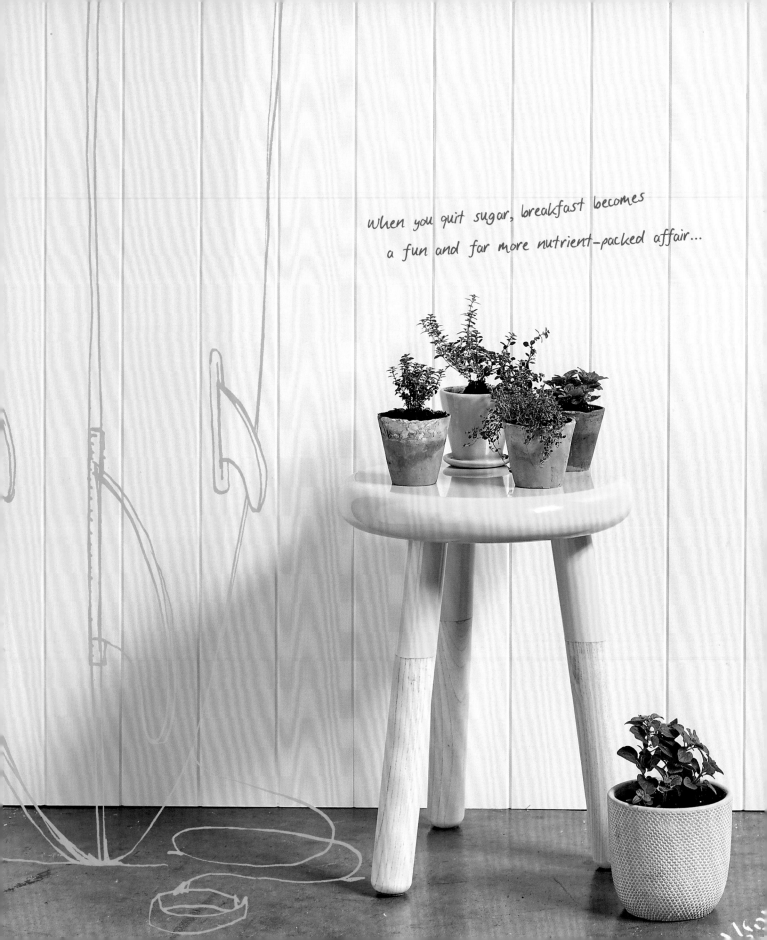

when you quit sugar, breakfast becomes
a fun and far more nutrient-packed affair...

A BUNCH OF INTERESTING BREAKFASTS

Dried, sugary flakes be gone!

STRAWBERRY AND AVOCADO TOASTIE

Toast the bread under the grill on one side only. Spread the untoasted side with the avocado, top with the strawberries and cheese, and toast under the grill until the cheese browns. Serve with plenty of pepper and the olive oil.

2 slices bread (preferably sourdough or
    gluten-free, if required)

½ avocado, mashed with a squeeze of lemon juice

¼ cup (40 g) strawberries, sliced

2 tablespoons soft goat's cheese

freshly ground black pepper, to taste

drizzle of olive oil

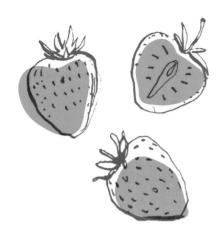

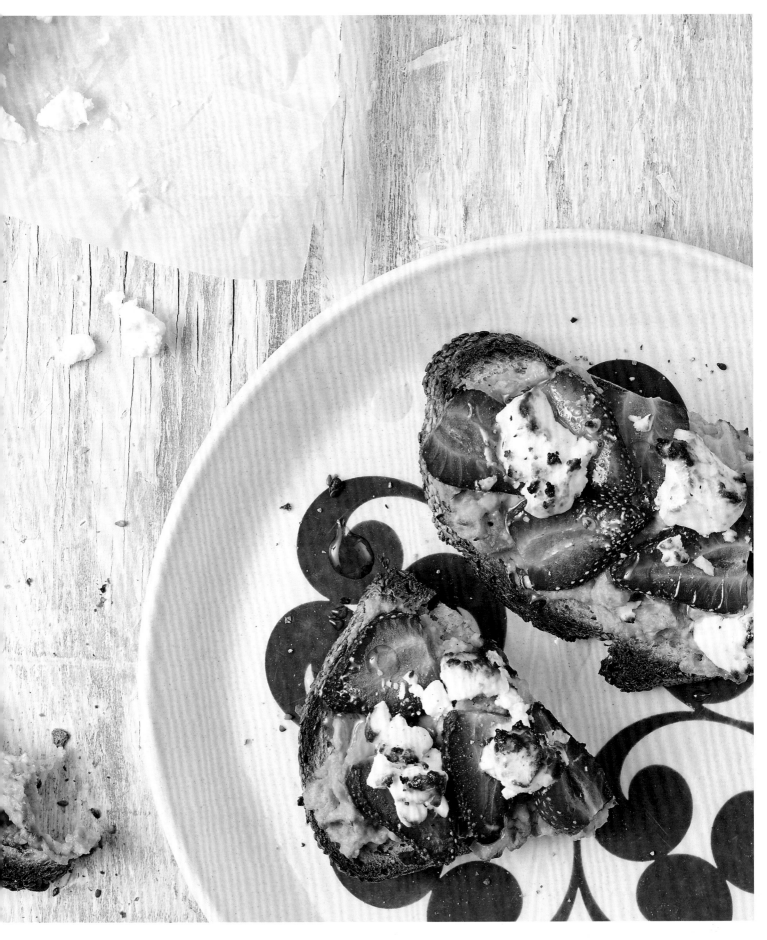

MEXICAN NACHO MEFFINS

A meffin is a muffin made with meat. You can choose to 'ice' these for impressive effect or keep them plain for easy toting.

Preheat the oven to 160°C (gas 3) and grease an 8-cup muffin tin. Heat the oil in a small frying pan over medium heat and sauté the onion until soft, about 3 minutes. Transfer the onion to a bowl, toss in the mince, eggs, Pumpkin Purée, corn kernels, crushed corn chips and spices, and season with a good pinch each of salt and pepper. Using your hands, mix well until all the ingredients are incorporated. Divide the mixture into 8 and press into the prepared muffin tin, pushing down firmly. Bake for 25 minutes, or until the meat is cooked through and the top is lightly browned. Remove from the oven and cool before serving.

Blend the avocado, Homemade Cream Cheese and citrus juice in a blender or using a stick blender, then dollop a tablespoonful on top of each meffin. Sprinkle with the remaining corn chips and chilli flakes.

NOTE: Meffins (without the 'icing') will keep in the fridge for 2–3 days or you can freeze them for 2–3 months.

2 teaspoons olive oil, plus extra for greasing

1 small onion, chopped

500 g lean organic beef mince

2 eggs

½ cup (125 ml) Pumpkin Purée (see page 51)

125 g can unsweetened corn kernels, drained

large handful of original (salted) corn chips, crushed

1 teaspoon ground cumin

1 teaspoon smoked sweet paprika

sea salt and freshly ground black pepper

1 small avocado

1 cup (225 g) Homemade Cream Cheese (see page 204)

1 tablespoon lemon or lime juice

chilli flakes (optional)

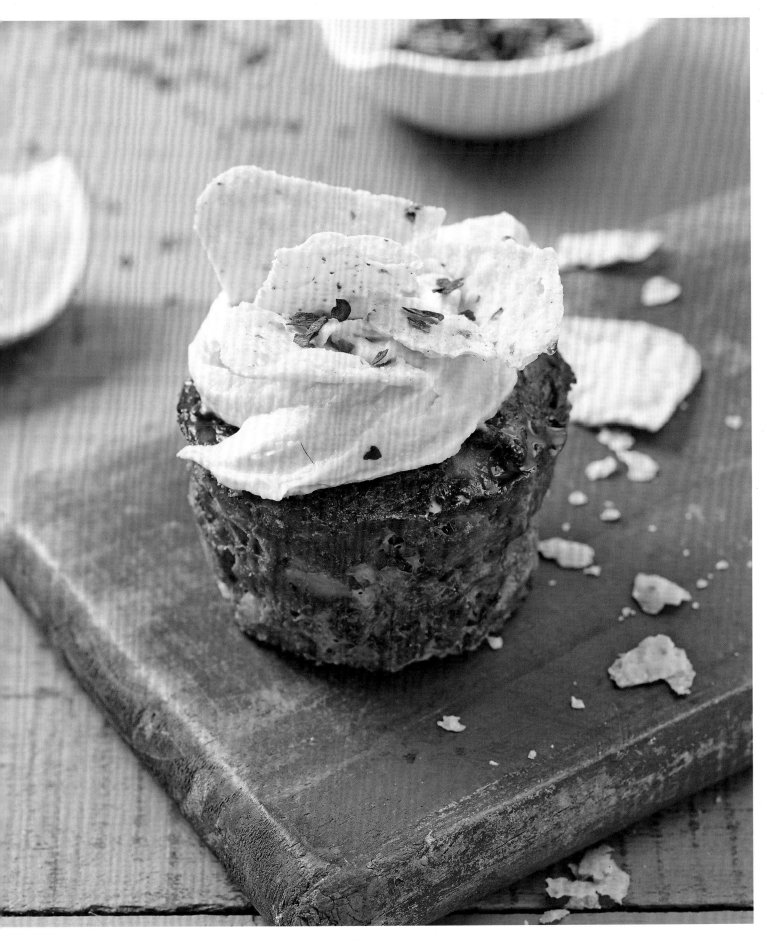

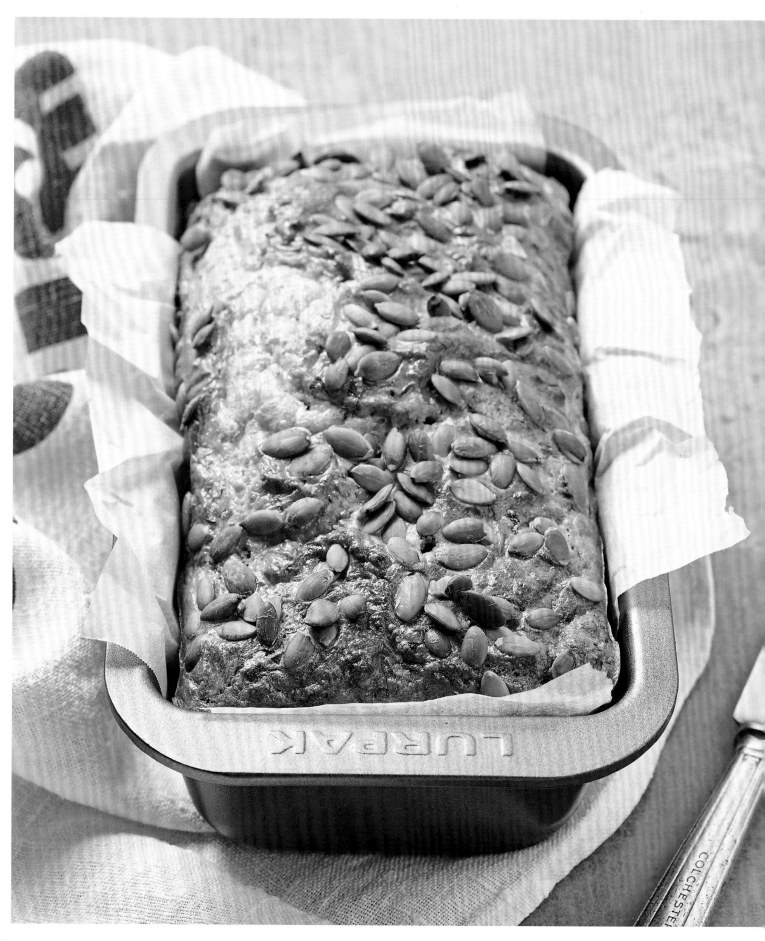

PALEO INSIDE-OUT BREAD

 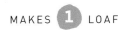

This simple loaf sees the outside sandwich toppers embedded in the bread. A meal-in-one in every slice.

Preheat the oven to 160°C (gas 3) and line a loaf tin with baking paper. In a large bowl, mix together the almond meal, arrowroot, salt and bicarbonate of soda. In a separate bowl and using a fork, whisk the eggs lightly with the apple cider vinegar. Add the parsley, olives, courgettes, ham and cheese and whisk well, then add the egg mix to the dry ingredients. Mix well to combine, then pour the dough into the prepared loaf tin and sprinkle with the pumpkin seeds.

Bake the bread for 30–35 minutes or until the top starts to turn golden and a skewer comes out clean. Remove from the oven and transfer to a wire rack. Allow to cool for 5 minutes before slicing. Freeze leftover slices between sheets of baking paper in a zip-lock bag.

Pimped Variation:
INSIDE-OUT FRENCH TOAST

Dip both sides of 2 slices in a mixture of 1 beaten egg and a dash of milk. Heat a little olive or coconut oil in a frying pan over medium–high heat and cook the egged bread for about 2 minutes on each side or until nicely browned. Serve with guacamole.

- 1½ cups (150 g) almond meal
- ¾ cup (100 g) arrowroot
- ½ teaspoon sea salt
- ½ teaspoon bicarbonate of soda
- 5 eggs
- 1½ teaspoons apple cider vinegar
- 1 tablespoon finely chopped flat-leaf parsley
- ⅓ cup (50 g) pitted olives, halved
- ¾ cup (125 g) grated courgettes
- ⅓ cup (50 g) finely diced ham
- ½ cup (50 g) finely grated parmesan cheese
- 2 tablespoons pumpkin seeds

NOT-QUITE-APPLE-CRUMBLE MUFFINS

I like to make these with chokos because, well, when they're in season they're dirt cheap. They're also very low in fructose. Otherwise, use apples, or peaches, which contain about a quarter the fructose of apples.

Preheat the oven to 180°C (gas 4) and line a 12-cup muffin tin with paper cases. In a large bowl, mix together the almond meal, arrowroot, baking powder, cinnamon and diced choko, peach or apple until the pieces are coated in the mixture. In another bowl or a measuring jug, mix the chia seeds with the water, ⅓ cup (75 ml) of the syrup and the vinegar until well combined.

Pour the chia mixture into the dry ingredients and fold through until just incorporated – do not over-mix or the muffins will lose their fluffiness – then spoon the batter into the prepared paper cases. Mix the chopped pecans with the remaining syrup and spoon on top of the batter.

Bake for 35–40 minutes or until the tops are starting to turn golden. Remove from the oven and cool on a wire rack.

NOTE: For an extra-indulgent way of serving these for dessert, try drizzling the muffins with Gooey Caramel Sauce (see page 140) and cream.

- 2½ (250 g) cups almond meal
- ¼ cup (30 g) arrowroot
- 2 teaspoons baking powder
- 2 teaspoons ground cinnamon
- 1 large choko, peeled and diced, or 2 peaches or green apples, diced
- 4 tablespoons chia seeds
- 1 cup (250 ml) water
- ½ cup (125 ml) rice malt syrup
- 1 tablespoon apple cider vinegar
- 1 cup (120 g) pecans, roughly chopped

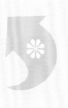

NEVER EATEN A CHOKO?

Also known as chayote or christophene, this squash-like vegetable may be found in some markets and West Indian shops. Simply peel it, steam it and eat the slippery little sucker with butter, pepper and salt, and serve as you would butternut squash.

NOURISHING KITCHERI

I was reminded of my love of this porridgy Indian staple when I was in London and ate the British Raj version of the dish (mostly called 'kedgeree') at The Wolseley. The original kitcheri ('mish-mash' in Hindi!) is an immensely healing Ayurvedic recipe said to be the most purifying and balancing dish conceivable. Based on basmati rice (the healthiest of the rices: low GI, densely nutritious and easiest to digest) and yellow split peas, or mung dal (huskless, therefore less phytic acid), it's a great source of protein, while the spices fire up digestion, removing toxins, particularly (say the Indian healers) pesticides and pollutants.

In a saucepan, warm the ghee and add the mustard seeds, cumin seeds, fennel seeds and ginger, and sauté for 1–2 minutes until the mustard seeds start to pop. Add split peas and rice and sauté for a few minutes, stirring.

Add the water, salt and ground spices to the pan and bring to the boil. Reduce the heat, then cover and cook until the peas and rice are tender (30–45 minutes). Serve with a squeeze of lime.

SOLO COOKERS: Freeze the remaining portions for up to 2 months. Or do a mini gut-resting 'fast' by eating it for breakfast and lunch for a couple of days in a row.

Serving Suggestions

Choose your garnish or extras according to your needs:

▶ Fresh coriander. Perfect for cooling Pitta.

▶ Coconut. Perfect for cooling Pitta and balancing Vata.

▶ Sweet potato. Add 1 cup (150 g), diced, 15 minutes after adding the water with an additional cup (250 ml) of water. Perfect for grounding Vata.

▶ Or top with a poached egg, a quartered boiled egg, smoked trout or haddock, or yoghurt.

Ingredients

- 2–3 tablespoons ghee
- 1 teaspoon black mustard seeds
- 1 teaspoon cumin seeds
- ½ teaspoon fennel seeds
- ½ tablespoon grated fresh ginger
- ⅔ cup (125 g) yellow split peas (mung dal), rinsed, soaked overnight and drained
- 1 cup (200 g) white basmati rice, rinsed well and drained
- 5 cups (1.2 litres) water
- 1 teaspoon rock salt
- 1 teaspoon ground cumin
- 1 teaspoon ground coriander
- 1 teaspooon ground turmeric
- ½ lime

THE FARTY THING

The Indians add asafoetida, a spice that tastes like garlic, to counteract the less desirable effect of the split peas. You can also cook the dish with a strip of the Japanese seaweed kombu. Either can be added to any kind of rice- or legume-based dish to reduce the chance of tummy upsets.

SARDINE BREAKFAST POTS

Preheat the oven to 180°C (gas 4). Press the spinach leaves into a small (1-cup/250 ml capacity) ovenproof ramekin or bowl and place the sardines on top. Break the eggs over the top and sprinkle with cheese. Place onto a baking tray and bake for 20 minutes.

SUSTAINABILITY TIP: It does seem a waste to turn on the oven for one little pot. Do a batch of Pumpkin or Sweet Potato Purée or Par-Cooked 'n' Frozen Beetroot (see page 51) – or any other dish that uses the oven at 180°C (gas 4) – while you're at it.

½ cup (15 g) baby spinach leaves

1–2 sardines, fresh and grilled (see page 116) or tinned and drained

2 eggs

4 tablespoons grated tasty cheese

SLOW-COOKED PORK BELLY BAKED BEANS

Great for breakfast, brunch or lunch with a fried or poached egg on top.

Rinse the soaked beans under cold running water, removing any discoloured ones, and toss into an electric slow cooker. Slice the pork belly into bite-sized pieces and add to the beans. Cover with the stock and add the paprika, oregano and pepper. Cook for 4 hours on high or 6 hours on low. The dish is ready to serve when beans are soft.

NOTE: If you don't have a slow cooker, you can use a heavy-based casserole pot instead, but add an extra cup (250 ml) of stock or water and reduce the cooking time to 1 hour, or until the beans are tender.

2 cups (340 g) dried borlotti or kidney beans, soaked overnight

400 g piece of pork belly, rind removed

4 cups (1 litre) Leftovers Chicken Stock (see page 191)

2 tablespoons smoked sweet paprika

1 tablespoon dried oregano

1 teaspoon freshly ground black pepper

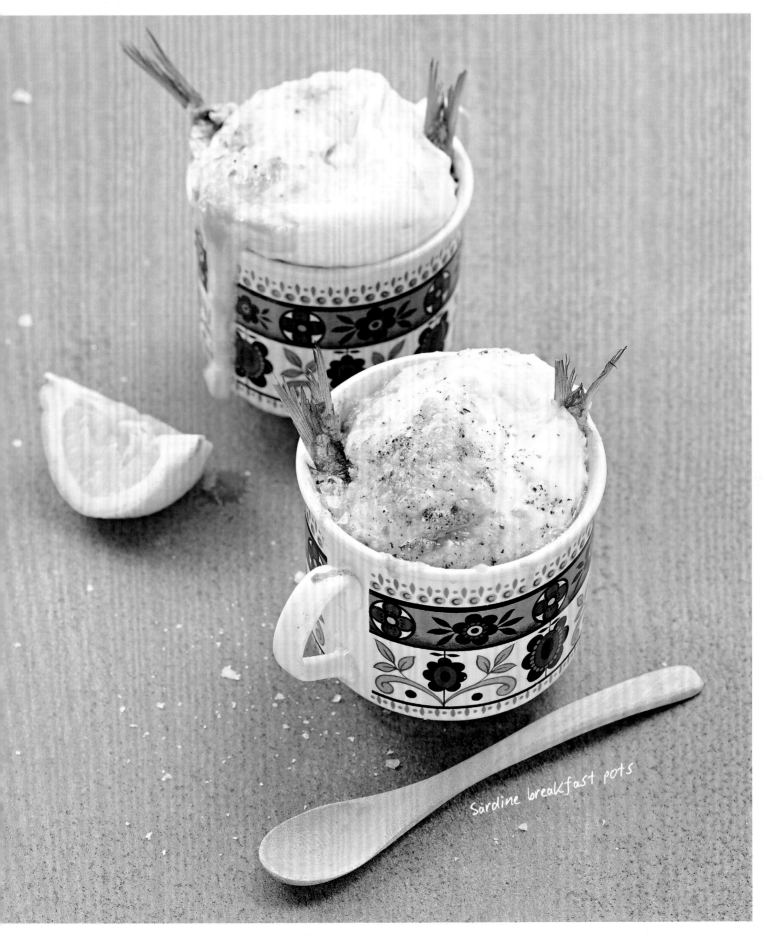

Sardine breakfast pots

PALEO CHOC-COCO MUGGIN

A muffin in a mug. Ergo, a muggin. Microwaves ain't great things, but my approach is this: if it's the difference between eating a decent breakfast and not, well, go for it. Sometimes it's the lesser of two evils.

Add all ingredients to a microwave-safe porcelain mug and mix with a spoon. Microwave on high for 1½–2 minutes. Serve with yoghurt.

NOTE: If you're carrying this to work, you can par-cook it first (so it doesn't spill).

¼ cup (25 g) almond meal or gluten-free self-raising flour

2 tablespoons desiccated coconut

1 tablespoon raw cacao powder

½ tablespoon rice malt syrup or ½ teaspoon granulated stevia

¼ cup (60 ml) coconut milk or any other type of milk

Greek-style full-fat organic plain yoghurt, to serve

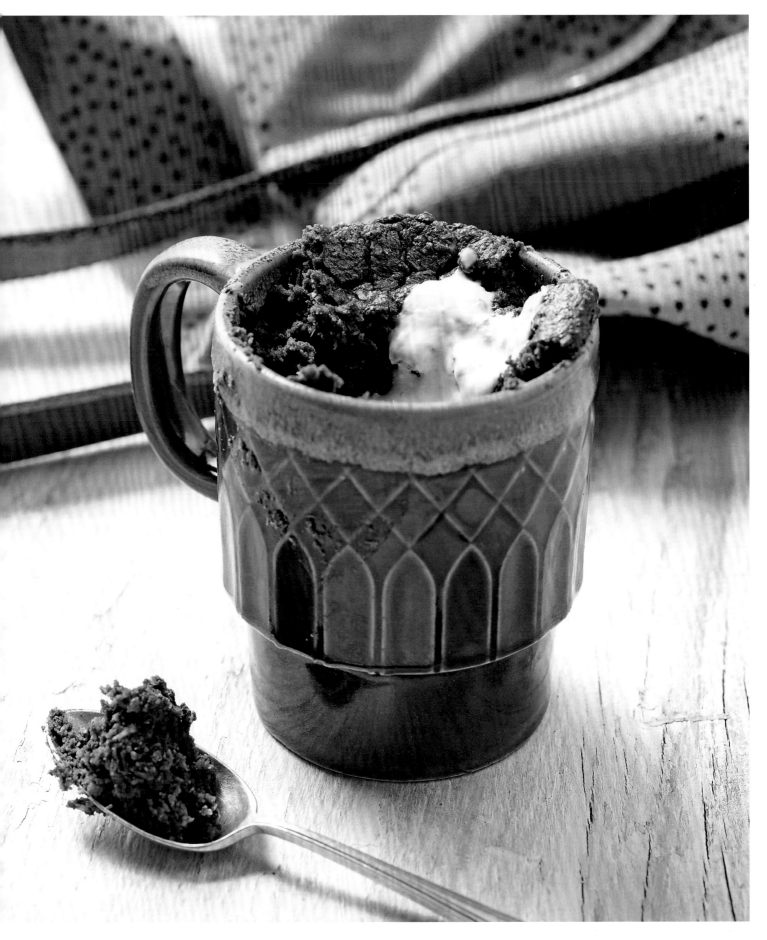

Breakfast in bed

BERRY OMELETTE

SERVES

This is the kind of Sunday Start to the Day I dream of a loved one serving me. With a pot of Earl Grey tea.

Separate the eggs and whisk the syrup and yolks with a stick blender. In a separate bowl, beat the egg whites until thick and fluffy, then fold into the yolk and syrup mixture.

Melt the butter in a 22-cm omelette pan over low heat. Pour in the eggs and sprinkle the berries over the top. Cook over low heat until the base is golden. Transfer the pan to your oven grill and brown very slightly. The omelette should be firm but a little creamy.

Serve with the mascarpone or yoghurt.

SOLO COOKERS: look out for individual-sized omelette pans (they exist) to make a solo serve. Note, however, you won't need to cook it as long in the smaller pan.

4 eggs

1–2 tablespoons rice malt syrup

1 tablespoon butter

1 cup (150 g) mixed berries (best fresh; if you use frozen, allow them to thaw and drain first)

mascarpone or full-fat organic plain yoghurt, to serve

RAW BREAKFAST BALLS

MAKES

In a large bowl, mix together the peanut butter, syrup, coconut cream and coconut oil. Add the salt, coconut flour and quinoa and mix to form a dough. Add a little more coconut flour if the mixture is too runny to form into balls. Pinch off bite-sized pieces of the dough and roll into walnut-sized balls. Roll each ball in the desiccated coconut to coat. Store in an airtight container and consume within 3 days.

Baked Variation:
PROTEIN COOKIES

Preheat the oven to 200°C (gas 6) and line a baking tray with baking paper. Flatten the previously prepared dough balls slightly and place on the prepared baking tray. Bake for 8 minutes or until the cookies are starting to turn golden. Remove from the oven and cool on a wire rack.

4 tablespoons natural, sugar-free and salt-free peanut butter

1 tablespoon rice malt syrup

½ cup (125 ml) coconut cream

¼ cup (50 g) coconut oil, melted

½ teaspoon sea salt

½ cup (50 g) coconut flour

⅓ cup (50 g) chilled cooked quinoa (see page 94)

½ cup (50 g) desiccated coconut, lightly toasted

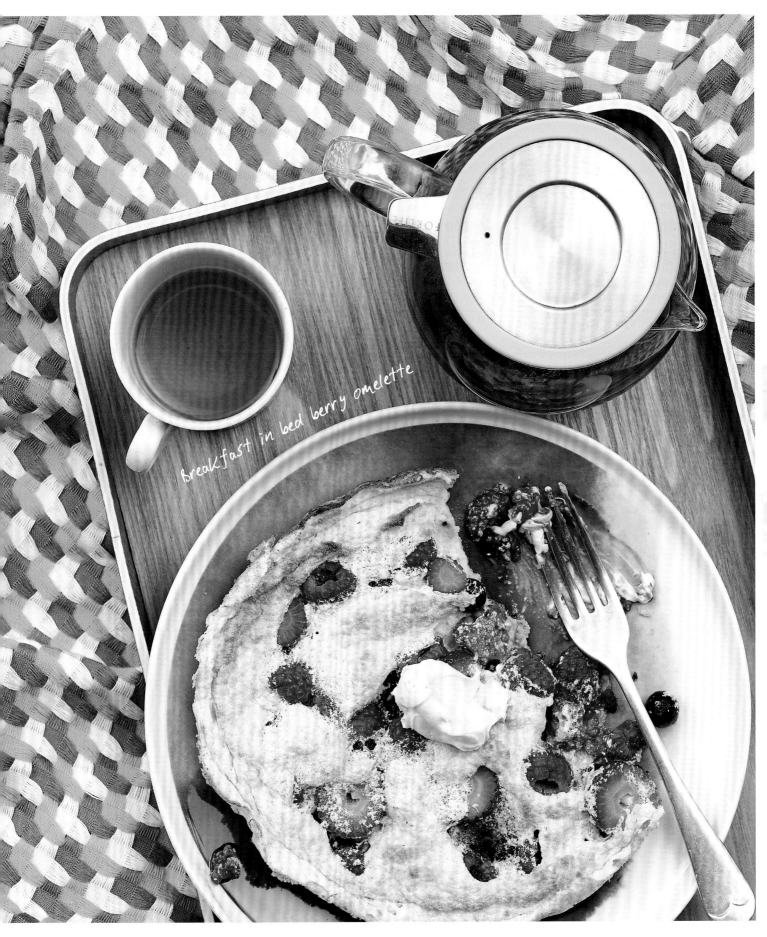

breakfast in bed berry omelette

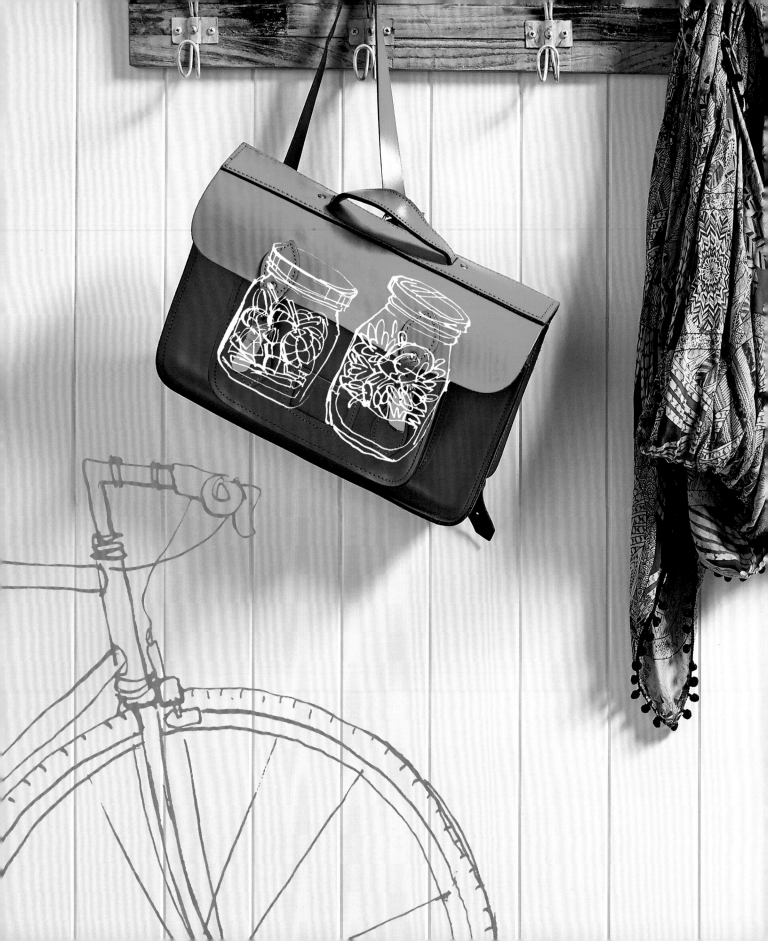

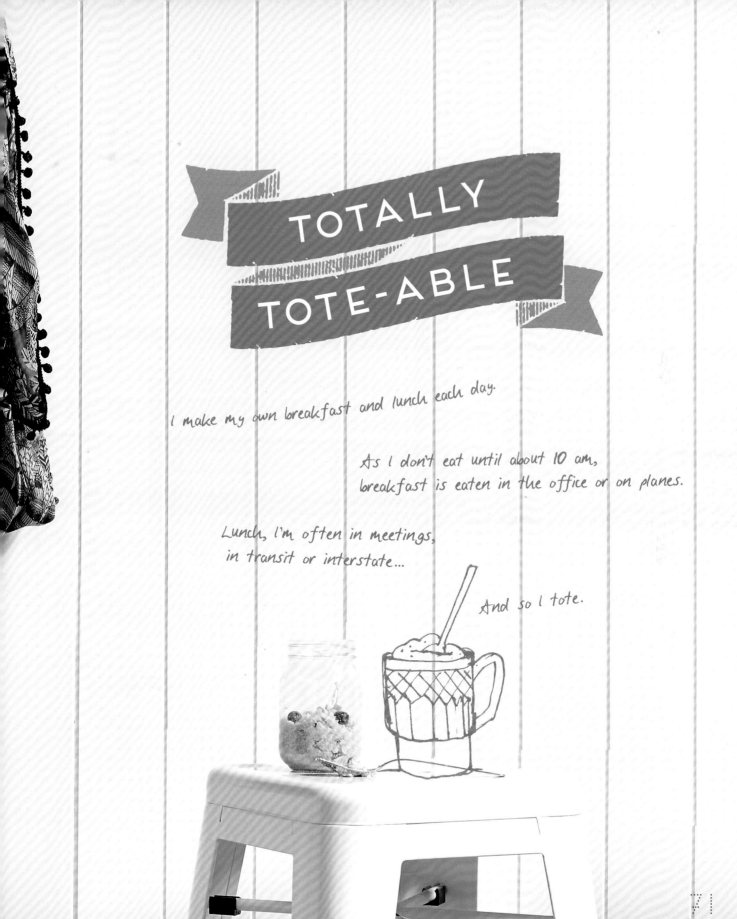

TOTALLY
TOTE-ABLE

I make my own breakfast and lunch each day.

As I don't eat until about 10 am,
breakfast is eaten in the office or on planes.

Lunch, I'm often in meetings,
in transit or interstate...

And so I tote.

CARROT CAKE PORRIDGE WHIP

OK, I've used half a banana here, but keep in mind it equates to a quarter of a banana per serve (about ¾ teaspoon of sugar). Not a huge deal. Agree?

Blend the oats, chia seeds, milk, vanilla, carrot, spices, salt, banana or avocado mix and the walnuts and coconut flakes until smooth. Pour into 2 jars and leave to soak overnight in the fridge, lids on. In the morning, top with yoghurt or Whipped Coconut Cream, granola and additional walnuts and coconut flakes.

THE BEAUTY OF OVERNIGHT OATS

Soaking your oats allows enzymes, lactobacilli and other helpful organisms to break down and neutralise the phytic acid in oats.

½ (50 g) cup rolled oats

1 tablespoon chia seeds (optional)

1½ cups (350 ml) coconut milk, including the cream on top (or any other kind of milk)

1 teaspoon vanilla extract or ¼ teaspoon vanilla powder

1 large carrot, finely grated (or just chopped roughly if using a high-speed blender)

1 teaspoon ground cinnamon

¼ teaspoon ground ginger

pinch each of ground nutmeg and sea salt

½ frozen banana or ½ avocado mixed with ½ tablespoon rice malt syrup

2 tablespoons crushed walnuts

2 tablespoons coconut flakes

yoghurt or Whipped Coconut Cream (see below)

additional walnuts, coconut flakes and sugar-free granola, to serve

WHIPPED COCONUT CREAM

This cream is a delight and can be used in place of icing by vegans and omnivores alike. It will keep in the fridge for up to a week.

Place the can of coconut cream in the fridge overnight upside down (be sure not to shake it beforehand). The next day, turn it the right way up and open the can without shaking it. Spoon out the top layer of liquid (keep this for smoothies or other recipes requiring coconut milk or coconut water). Leave the rest of the harder cream in the can, add the stevia, then blend using a stick blender until thick and creamy. (If you don't have a stick blender, remove the cream from the can and whip using a bench or hand mixer or in a blender.) For the best texture, refrigerate for at least 2 hours before serving. The longer it is refrigerated, the thicker the cream gets.

400 ml can coconut cream

1 tablespoon granulated stevia

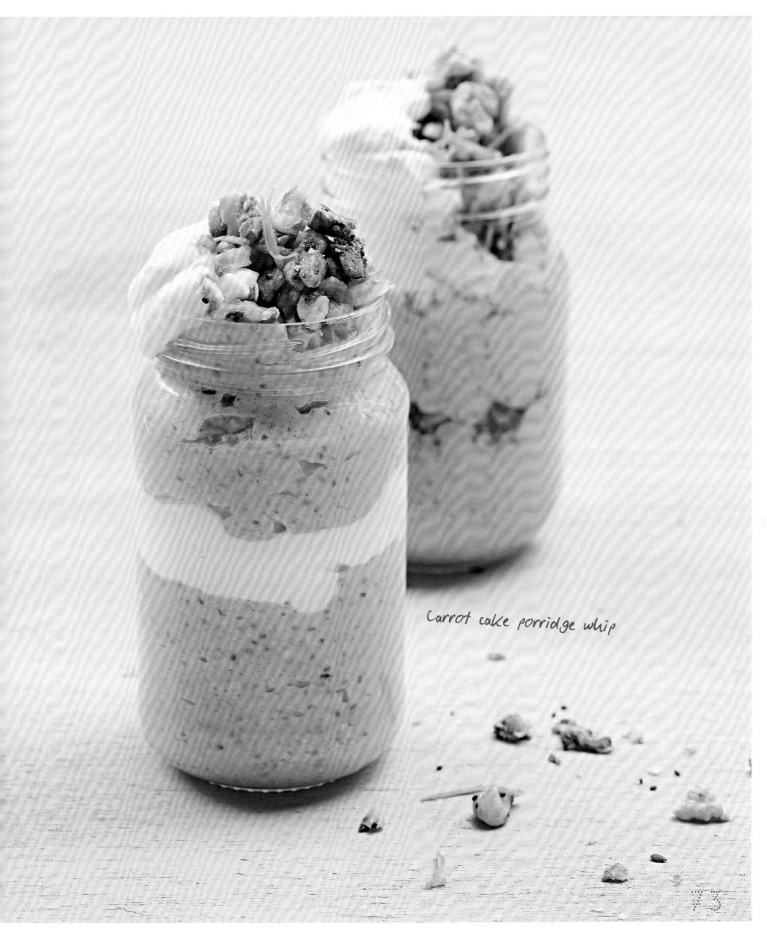

Carrot cake porridge whip

SNICKERY PUMPKIN MUD SMOOTHIE

SERVES 2

This smoothie is a full and nutritious breakfast experience. Depending on how muddy or smooth you like your smoothie, you may wish to add some extra milk, water or ice.

Throw all the ingredients into a blender and blend until smooth. If you're using a high-powered blender, add the ice. Serve in a glass jar or a large insulated KeepCup.

small handful of baby spinach leaves

1½ tablespoons raw cacao powder (or to taste)

½ (125 ml) cup milk (any kind, including coconut) or full-fat organic plain yoghurt

1 tablespoon vanilla protein powder (you can use a vegan, legume-protein-based powder or a whey-based version – just ensure it has no sugar)

1 tablespoon natural, sugar- and salt-free crunchy peanut butter

½ teaspoon five-spice mix or a combination of ground cinnamon, nutmeg and ginger

½ cup (125 ml) Pumpkin Purée (see page 51)

pinch of sea salt

small handful of ice (optional)

MOCHA TOBLERONE THICKSHAKE

SERVES 2

Blitz the whole hazelnuts in a blender. Follow the instructions for the Snickery Pumpkin Mud Smoothie (above), but omit the pumpkin, replace the peanut butter with the hazelnuts and add the black coffee.

2 tablespoons whole hazelnuts

½ cup (125 ml) black coffee

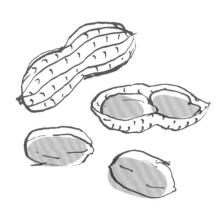

HOT TURMERIC MILKSHAKE

Enjoy this pacifying beverage on windy, unbalanced days when your Vata energy is out of whack. There's no need to add stevia or syrup to this lovely earthing drink, although 1 teaspoon of coconut oil will add enough sweetness if you're after some.

Throw the almonds and milk into a blender and blend until smooth. Stir through the spices. Pour into 2 glass jars and heat in a microwave gently to serve.

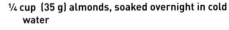

¼ cup (35 g) almonds, soaked overnight in cold water

1 cup (250 ml) milk (any kind, including coconut)

¼ teaspoon ground or – better – fresh, grated turmeric

1 teaspoon ground cinnamon

1 teaspoon ground ginger

1 teaspoon vanilla powder

PEANUT BUTTER 'N' JELLY PORRIDGE WHIP

MAKES 2

Throw the oats, chia seeds, milk, protein powder and vanilla into a blender and blend until smooth. Pour into 2 jars, put the lids on and leave to soak overnight in the fridge, lids on. Using a stick blender on a low speed, add the peanut or almond butter to the Whipped Coconut Cream ½ tablespoon at time. Add the syrup and blend a little more, then store in the fridge overnight. In the morning top with the strawberry jam and the peanut butter whip.

NOTE: You can make the peanut butter whip in bulk using the whole quantity of Whipped Coconut Cream, 3–4 tablespoons peanut butter and 2 teaspoons rice malt syrup. It will keep in the fridge for a week (although you might need to rewhip it to get it fluffy again).

½ cup (50 g) uncooked rolled oats

1 tablespoon chia seeds

1½ cups (350 ml) milk (any kind)

2 tablespoons vanilla protein powder

1 teaspoon vanilla extract or ¼ teaspoon vanilla powder

1 tablespoon peanut butter or almond butter

½ cup (120 ml) Whipped Coconut Cream (see page 72)

1 teaspoon rice malt syrup

1 tablespoon Strawberry Jam (see page 207)

CHEAT'S OPTION

Add some coconut flakes before soaking overnight, skip the peanut butter whip step and simply top the porridge with fresh or frozen strawberries, a dollop of peanut butter and some walnuts or pecans, then heat in the microwave once you're at work and eat with plain yoghurt.

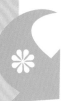

FOUR WAYS to have a Green Glowin' Skin Smoothie

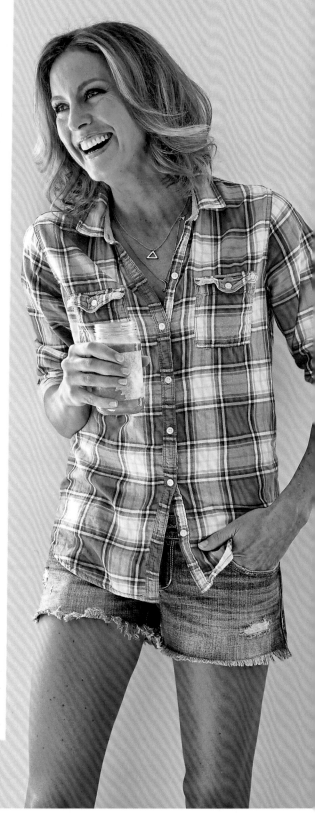

There are many ways to skin a cucumber and make yourself a cleansing green juice. I have my principles, however.

I blend or purée; I 'juice' using a blender not a juicer. That is, I blitz and consume the whole vegetable and fruit, rather than extract the juice only. I throw in pips and all (and a little zest from lemons and limes – they're said to be cancer-fighting). Fibre is important, especially if you're using a little fruit or high-fructose vegetables. Besides, tossing out the fibre is a bad case of food wastage. Making my smoothies this way also means I don't need an expensive juicer to clutter my kitchen.

I use a high-powered blender, although a regular blender will do the job, too. If using the former, add extra ice (and place it, along with hard veggies, in the blender first). If using the latter, stick to softer greens like cucumber, lettuce, baby spinach and watercress.

I incorporate some fat – avocado, coconut, milk and/or chia seeds. The goodness from green vegetables is best absorbed with fat so it's a bad case of wasted vitamins if you don't have a little in the mix. **The most important vitamins in vegetables – A, E, D and K – are only absorbed when eaten with fat.** I also try to incorporate some protein, to make my cup floweth over and become a full meal.

Place the ingredients in the blender in the order listed, and add water as required. Blend until smooth (not too long as it will heat the greens) and divide between 2 glass jars with lids, or insulated KeepCups.

*Wrap your laughing gear around
a few of the combinations opposite.*

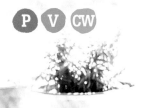

P V CW

1. SWEET, CLEAN PROTEIN MACHINE

This one's a meal-in-a-cup. Kids and blokes are fans.

Ice, 3 frozen strawberries, 1 peeled kiwifruit, 3 handfuls of lettuce/baby spinach/watercress/rocket (whatever's to hand), 4 tablespoons vanilla protein powder, large handful of mint, 1 teaspoon chia seeds (optional), 1 cup (250 ml) coconut water.

2. I AM GRACEFUL (ANTI-INFLAMMATORY BLEND)

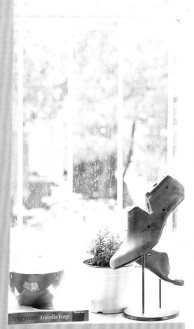

This is my go-to refresher when my auto-immune disease is playing up.

Ice, 1 tablespoon chia seeds, 1 large cucumber, 1 lemon, ½ green apple, 2 celery stalks, handful of coriander, 3-cm knob each of fresh ginger and turmeric (if available), 1 cup (250 ml) coconut water, pinch of granulated stevia or a few drops of liquid stevia (optional).

3. THE MAGNIFICENT (SAVOURY CLEANSER)

This one is an acquired taste. Some find it an odd concept if they're not used to savoury drinks . . . Bloody Mary fans will warm to the idea, however.

Ice, ½ (75 g) cup chopped fennel (or 2 celery stalks), 3-cm knob each of fresh ginger and turmeric (if available), handful of baby spinach, watercress or rocket (whatever's on hand), 1 small soft avocado, ½ pepper (red, yellow or orange is best), 1 cup (225 g) Par-Cooked 'n' Frozen broccoli, big handful of flat-leaf parsley and/or coriander, 1 tablespoon chopped red onion, 1 lime (including some of the zest), 1 cup (250 ml) coconut water (or water), big pinch of cayenne pepper (or chilli powder or a dash of Tabasco), good grind of salt, pinch of granulated stevia.

4. THE SUCCULENT (BERRY GUT CLEANSER)

For restoring good metabolism with a berries 'n' cream vibe.

Ice, 2 handfuls of baby spinach, 1 cup (150 g) frozen mixed berries, 1 cup (250 ml) kefir or full-fat organic plain yoghurt or almond milk (with ½ cup (50 g) almond meal), 2 tablespoons coconut flakes or coconut oil (added at the end so it doesn't go cold and hard), 2 tablespoons whey (optional), pinch of granulated stevia.

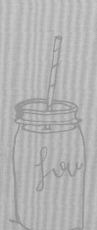

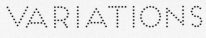

VARIATIONS

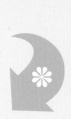

► Feel free to throw in other greenery, if you have it lying around: celery, cucumber, fennel, pak choi, Par-Cooked 'n' Frozen broccoli or kale (see page 51), lettuce (any kind).

► Invest in a sugar-free green powder (a mix of dehydrated greens) and add a tablespoon to any of the combos.

Some handy tips for making

THINGS IN JARS

You'll notice many of the tote-ables serve 2.
One for today, one for tomorrow (to save time + bother).

The ADDED BONUS OF FREEZING
YOUR SOUP in a JAR:

IT MAKES YOUR TOTE-ABLE
TOTALLY UNSPILLABLE

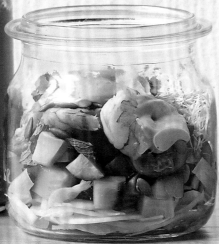

SNICKERY PUMPKIN
MUD SMOOTHIE

CLEAN OUT,
COOL DOWN
WATERCRESS
SOUP

USE A BROAD-MOUTHED JAR
FOR YOUR SALADS

[so you can fit
your fork in]

ANOTHER ANTI-SPILLAGE TRICK:

ADD CHIA SEEDS TO YOUR WHIP OR
SMOOTHIE TO MAKE THINGS BUDGE-PROOF.

You can always add extra
milk or water to serve.

CHOCOLATE COCO-NUTTY
GRANOLA CLUSTERS
with YOGHURT.

I MAKE SURE I DRINK GREEN
SMOOTHIES WITH SOME
SORT OF PROTEIN AND FAT
[a boiled egg or two,
or some nuts so
the fat is absorbed].

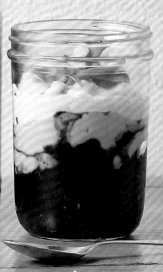

I AM GRACEFUL
(ANTI-INFLAMMATORY
BLEND) GREEN
GLOWIN' SKIN
SMOOTHIE

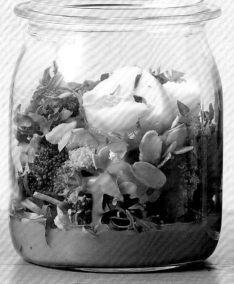

IF YOU'RE GOING TO DUMP YOUR SALAD-
IN-A-JAR INTO A BOWL TO SERVE,

put your dressing or sauce
on the bottom of the jar

[so that when you tip it,
it winds up on top!]

ICELANDIC
SKYR PARFAIT

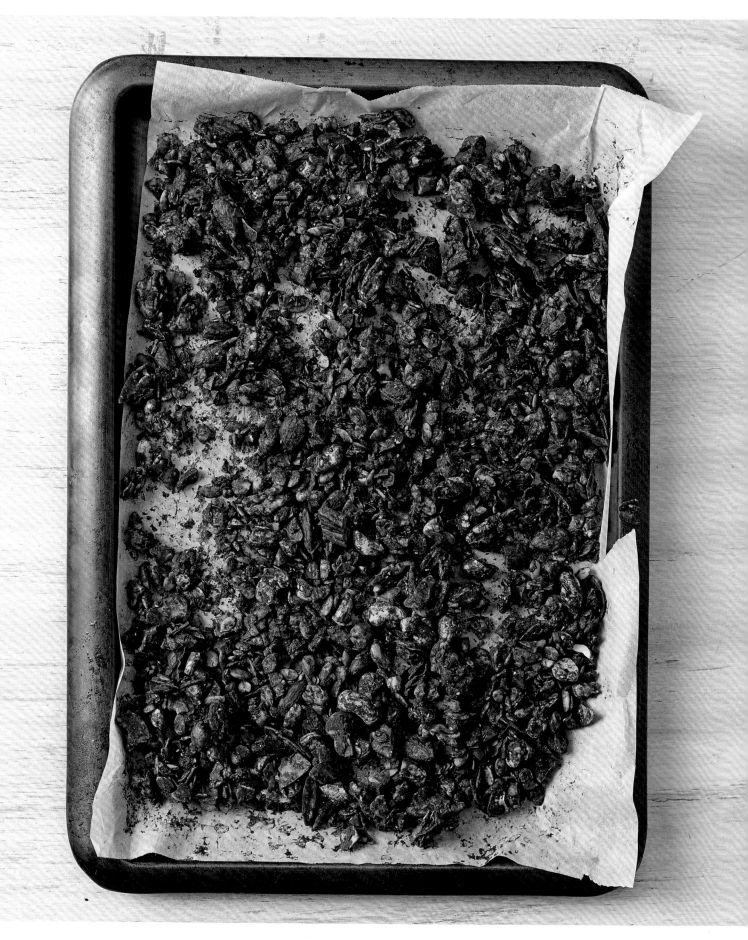

CHOCOLATE COCO-NUTTY GRANOLA CLUSTERS

 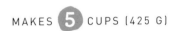

These globules of goodness work for breakfast, as a snack and for dessert. You can choose to omit or reduce the amount of rice malt syrup to taste. I personally find the coconut oil provides enough sweetness.

Preheat the oven to 120°C (gas ½) and line a baking tray with baking paper. Combine all the ingredients except the yoghurt, then spread evenly on the prepared tray. Bake for 15–20 minutes or until golden, turning halfway through the cooking time. I like to bake mine until it's quite dark – the darker, the crunchier. Remove from the oven and allow to cool.

To serve, spoon the yoghurt into a glass jar or bowl and top with ½ cup (85 g) of clusters.

NOTE: This makes a great dessert too. You can also try sprinkling on some Whipped Coconut Cream (see page 72).

3 cups (175 g) coconut flakes

2 cups (250 g) mixed almonds, cashews, pecans, walnuts and pumpkin seeds (preferably activated, see page 204), roughly chopped

2 tablespoons chia seeds

1 teaspoon ground cinnamon (optional)

80–100 g coconut oil or melted butter

4 tablespoons rice malt syrup (optional)

½ cup (50 g) raw cacao powder

2 tablespoons cacao nibs

½ cup (125 ml) Greek-style full-fat organic plain yoghurt or unsweetened coconut yoghurt, to serve

FIVE WAYS *with Great Grated Salad*

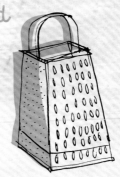

I make this two-step salad and keep it in the fridge for a few days, adding different dressings, flavours and protein on demand (perfect for Solo Cookers!).

Any salad I don't finish, I turn into fritters by adding some chia seeds or arrowroot (to soak up the liquid) and an egg or two, forming into patties and frying, or throw in a soup.

BASIC GREAT GRATED SALAD

SERVES **4**

Grate the carrots, courgettes and cauliflower or swede. Use a blender with a grater attachment, if possible; that way you can simply add the rest of the ingredients to the blender bowl. Stir through the spring onions or onion and divide among 4 large, broad glass jars. Top each salad with the dressing of choice and the seeds.

Now try these 'build on' variations, opposite.

2 carrots

2 small courgettes

1 cup (225 g) cauliflower florets or 1 swede

4 spring onions or 1 red onion, finely chopped

a dressing of your choice
    (see recipes on page 205)

½ cup (75 g) pumpkin seeds and/or sunflower seeds, lightly toasted (toasting is optional)

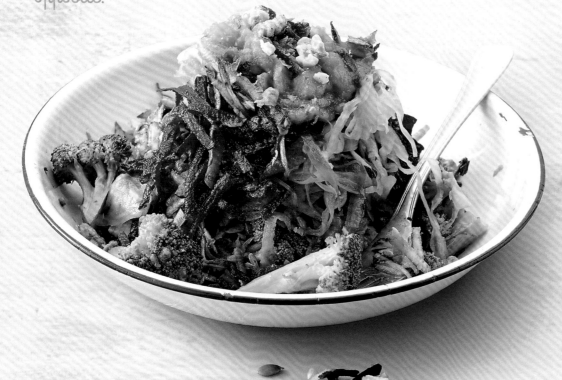

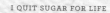

1. VIETNAMESE CHICKEN *Great Grated Salad*

Add: leftover chicken from Crispy Roast Chook (see page 111), sliced red pepper and mint leaves.
Swap: sesame seeds for the pumpkin seeds.
Dressing: Take-Me-Anywhere Asian Dressing (see page 205) or Korean Mayo (see page 209).

2. RAINBOW *Great Grated Salad*

Add: grated beetroot and crumbled soft feta.
Swap: lightly toasted walnuts for the pumpkin seeds, whole Par-Cooked 'n' Frozen broccoli (page 51) for the cauliflower.
Dressing: Dressing in a Jar (see page 205) or Pumpkin Purée (page 51).

3. ALKALISING *Great Grated Salad*

Add: defrosted Par-Cooked 'n' Frozen broccoli florets (see page 51), cut into very small pieces, and sprouts (see page 162) or Homemade Sauerkraut (see page 200).
Dressing: Creamy Green Detox Sauce (see page 209) or Alkalising Potion (see page 205).

4. NIÇOISE *Great Grated Salad*

Add: 95 g can tuna (in brine, sustainably fished), cherry tomatoes, cut into quarters, chopped anchovies, basil leaves, salt and freshly ground black pepper; feel free to add a boiled egg.
Dressing: Tartare Sauce (see page 208) or A-Little-Bit-Frenchy Dressing (see page 205).

5. PRAWN COCKTAIL MISH-MASH *Great Grated Salad*

Add: watercress, alfalfa/radish shoots or roughly chopped rocket leaves, ¼ cucumber or avocado, diced, 3 cherry tomatoes, cut into quarters, and 80 g cooked peeled prawns.
Swap: ⅓ cup (50 g) very finely sliced fennel for some of the grated vegetables and a few mint leaves for the spring onions.
Dressing: Thousand Island Dressing (see page 209).

VARIATIONS

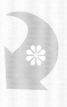

▶ Grated pumpkin instead of grated carrot.

▶ Grated radish or celeriac instead of cauliflower.

▶ Try a 'hot salad': heat in a microwave (be sure to remove metal or plastic jar lids beforehand). This works well when you add an egg on top.

ICELANDIC SKYR PARFAIT

When I was travelling in Iceland, checking out their Slow Food scene, I embraced the traditional skyr that's served for breakfast, lunch (on sandwiches) and after dinner (with berries, instead of ice cream). It's a cultured cheese brimful of beneficial gut bacteria that's pretty similar to the Homemade Cream Cheese I've been making for years. I've borrowed this lovely breakfast mousse presentation from the Aldin café in downtown Reykjavik, a place where locals knit beanies over their steaming coffee in the morning before work. As you do when you live in Iceland.

Throw the avocado and three-quarters of the coconut milk into a bowl and blend using a stick blender. In a separate bowl, blend the rest of the coconut milk with the cream cheese. Layer the berries, cream cheese and avocado mousse in 2 large jars and sprinkle with the coconut shavings.

SOLO COOKERS: The extra serve will keep in the fridge for a day or two.

½ **avocado**

1 cup (250 ml) **coconut milk**

½ cup (115 g) **Homemade Cream Cheese (see page 204)**

½ cup (75 g) **frozen berries, heated in a small saucepan for a few minutes, then cooled**

coconut shavings, lightly toasted

UP 'N' GO BREAKFAST WHIP

Packaged liquid-breakfasts-in-boxes are nutritional travesties, containing huge amounts of toxic seed oils (yes!), sugar and chemicals. Make your own instead. Teenage boys – nay, blokes of all ages – seem to really like this one.

Place all the ingredients in a high-powered blender and blend until smooth. Serve in a glass jar with a lid.

2–3 **Weetabix (or any low-sugar wheat breakfast biscuit), crushed**

⅓ cup (75 ml) **milk of your choice**

2 **ice cubes**

½ tablespoon **rice malt syrup (optional)**

1 tablespoon **almond butter or vanilla protein powder**

2 **frozen strawberries**

CLEAN OUT, COOL DOWN WATERCRESS SOUP

SERVES **2**

To eat watercress is to really give your insides a thorough scrub and polish. It contains all essential vitamins and is extremely alkalising. Wait! There's more. It's rich in fatty acids, chlorophyll and iodine . . . a boon when you're detoxing. When, according to Ayurvedic tradition, your Pitta energy is a bit worked up, which can happen in summer, or when inflammation is rife from digestive stress, the cooling, alkalising properties of this soup will get you back on track. You can serve it hot or cold, but make sure you include a little saturated fat – via the cream or yoghurt – to ensure you absorb all those minerals and vitamins.

Heat the butter in a saucepan over low heat and sauté the onion until soft. Add the stock and potato. Bring to the boil, then simmer until the potatoes are soft, about 20 minutes. Add the watercress, season with salt and pepper, add the cumin and cayenne pepper, and stir for 3 minutes. Remove from the heat and purée in batches in a blender or using a stick blender. If you care about keeping the vibrant green of the watercress, after blending, pour the soup into a metal bowl and place it in a sink full of ice-cold water. Pour into glass jars with lids and serve hot or cold with a swirl of the cream or yoghurt.

SOLO COOKERS: Freeze extra portions in the jars.

NOTE: The added bonus of freezing your Soup in a Jar: it makes your tote-able totally spill-free. This is a summer soup, but if you're making it in cooler times, feel free to replace the onion with leek.

Green(er) Variation:
POTATO-FREE WATERCRESS SOUP

If you want to make this soup even cleaner, replace the potato with fennel or cauliflower. Or omit altogether and add one soft avocado instead, once the soup has cooled but before you purée it. You can also choose to sweat the onion in a little stock rather than butter.

1 tablespoon butter

1 onion, finely chopped

5 cups (1.2 litres) Leftovers Chicken Stock (see page 191)

1 red potato, diced

2–3 large bunches of watercress, chopped

salt and freshly ground black pepper, to taste

½ teaspoon ground cumin

¼ teaspoon cayenne pepper

double cream or full-fat organic plain yoghurt, to serve

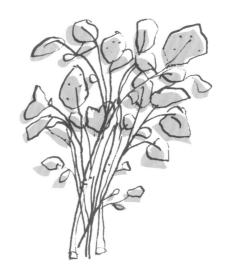

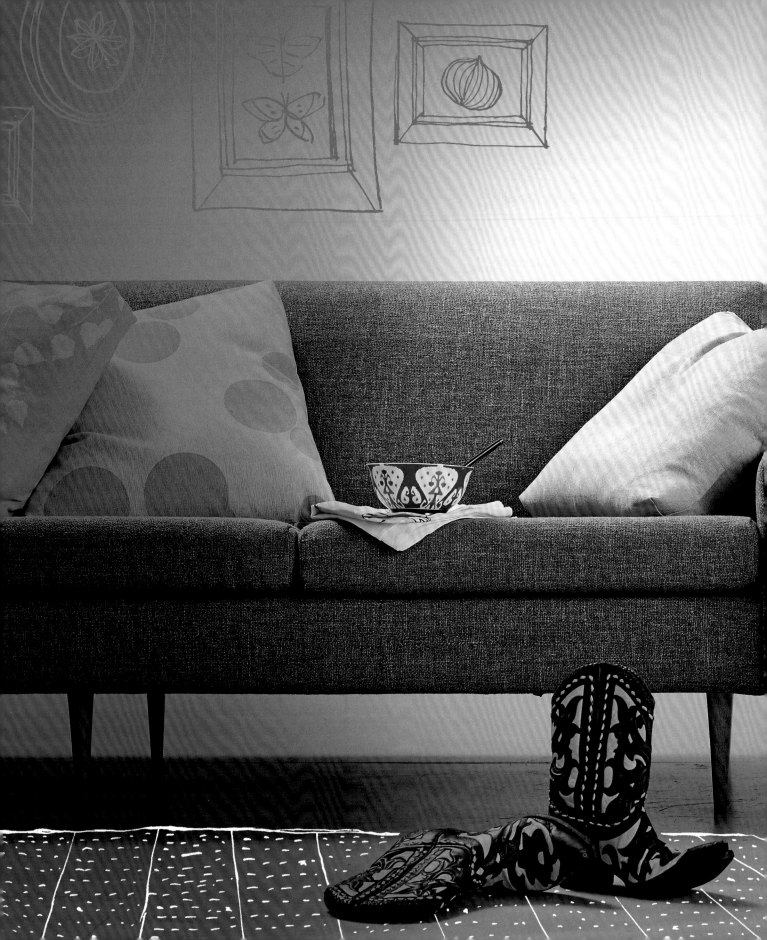

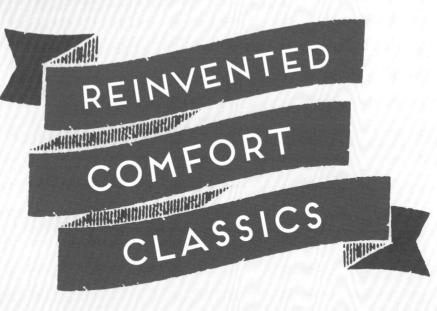

REINVENTED COMFORT CLASSICS

This is the section where I take the meals that everyone loves (but wishes could be healthier) and redo them with a same-same-but-sustainable-and-nutrient-dense twirl.

PS I've thrown in a few kids' and blokes' favourites for good measure.

DECONSTRUCTED HAMBURGER
in a bowl

 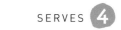

This dish essentially takes the best bits of a burger and dumps them in a bowl, as an artsy salad creation. I like to make this quite a roughed-up salad and crumble the patties a little. You might, too.

To make the patties, combine the mince, onion and parsley in a large bowl, season to taste and mix well using your hands. Divide the mixture into 4 even-sized patties. Heat the oil, butter or ghee in a frying pan over medium heat. Cook the patties on both sides, for 5–8 minutes in total. Sprinkle the cheese on top and cover the pan for a couple of minutes to allow the patties to cook through and the cheese to melt.

Meanwhile, divide the rocket, carrot and avocado among 4 bowls. Remove the patties from the pan and place one on top of each salad. Turn the heat to low and cook the onion in the meat juices. Take a good 5 minutes or so to 'sweat' the onion, so it caramelises a little. Deglaze with the vinegar before the onion catches, then add the thyme and cook a little longer, until the onion is very soft. Add to the bowls. Finally, toss the beetroot in the same pan to heat through. Remove and place on top of salads. Stir a swirl of harissa through the yoghurt, then serve the salads with the yoghurt, mustard and sauerkraut or cucumbers.

SOLO COOKERS: Freeze 3 of the patties (before cooking them) and adjust the remaining ingredients to suit.

Optional Extras:

▸ WHEY-GOOD MAYO
(see page 208)

▸ HALVED CHERRY TOMATOES

▸ BEETROOT AND APPLE RELISH
(see page 199) instead of the beetroot.

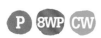

PATTIES
600 g lean organic beef mince

1 small onion

½ tablespoon chopped flat-leaf parsley

sea salt and freshly ground black pepper

1 tablespoon coconut oil, butter or ghee

1 cup (100 g) grated cheese

SALAD
4 large handfuls of rocket leaves

2 carrots, grated

1 avocado, diced

1 large onion, sliced

1 tablespoon apple cider vinegar

½ teaspoon dried thyme,
   or a few sprigs of thyme

2 cups (300 g) Par-Cooked 'n' Frozen
   beetroot (see page 51), thawed

ACCOMPANIMENTS
2 tablespoons harissa paste or
   1 tablespoon harissa powder mixed
   with a little water and olive oil

1 cup (250 ml) full-fat organic plain
   yoghurt

mustard

Homemade Sauerkraut (see page 200) or
   Fermented Cucumbers (see page 199)

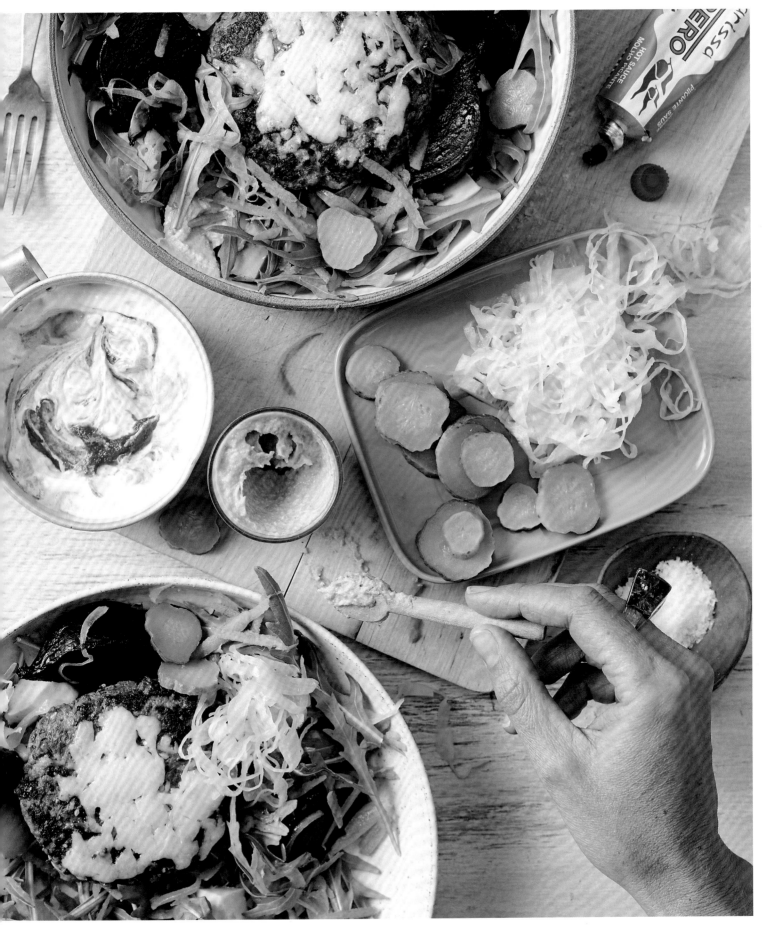

The great thing about this take on the fast-food fave is it allows you to use fish offcuts (you're pulverising the fish, so why waste a fillet!). Instead of bream you can use any type of firmer white fish, such as skinless mahi mahi fillets. Or whichever white fish your fishmonger has as offcuts.

Preheat the oven to 200°C (gas 6) and line a baking tray with baking paper. Cut the sweet potatoes in half crossways, then cut lengthways into 1-cm slices. Cut the slices into medium-chunk fries. Pat dry with kitchen paper, then toss in the oil. Spread out on the prepared baking tray, leaving room for the fish fingers, and pop in the oven for about 10 minutes.

Meanwhile, make the fish fingers by blitzing the fish with the egg in a food processor or using a stick blender, in batches if required. Transfer to a bowl and add the chives, salt and pepper. Mix well, using a spoon. Measure out 4 tablespoons of the fish mixture at a time and form into 8 tight logs using your hands – latex-free gloves are helpful here! Coat each log in the parmesan. Remove the baking tray from the oven and add the fish fingers. Return to the oven and bake for 20–25 minutes, turning the logs halfway through, until the parmesan is golden and the fish fingers are cooked through. Serve with the slaw or celery heart salad, and Tartare Sauce.

SOLO COOKERS: You can freeze the cooked fish fingers for up to 2 months.

- 2 medium sweet potatoes
- 1 tablespoon olive oil or coconut oil, melted
- 600 g sustainable bream fillets or preferably offcuts
- 1 egg
- 1 tablespoon chopped chives (dried are OK too)
- ½ teaspoon sea salt
- 1 teaspoon freshly ground black pepper
- ½ cup (50 g) coarsely grated parmesan cheese
- Slaw (see page 92) or Sardinian Celery Heart Salad (see page 192) and Tartare Sauce (see page 208), to serve

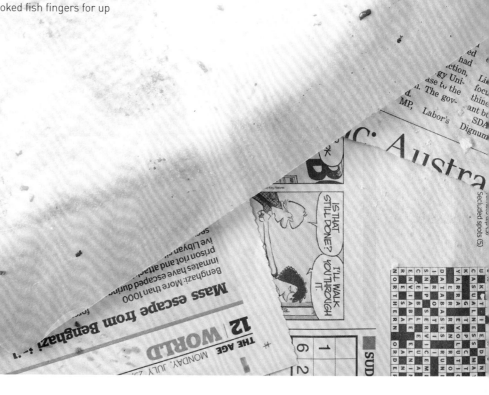

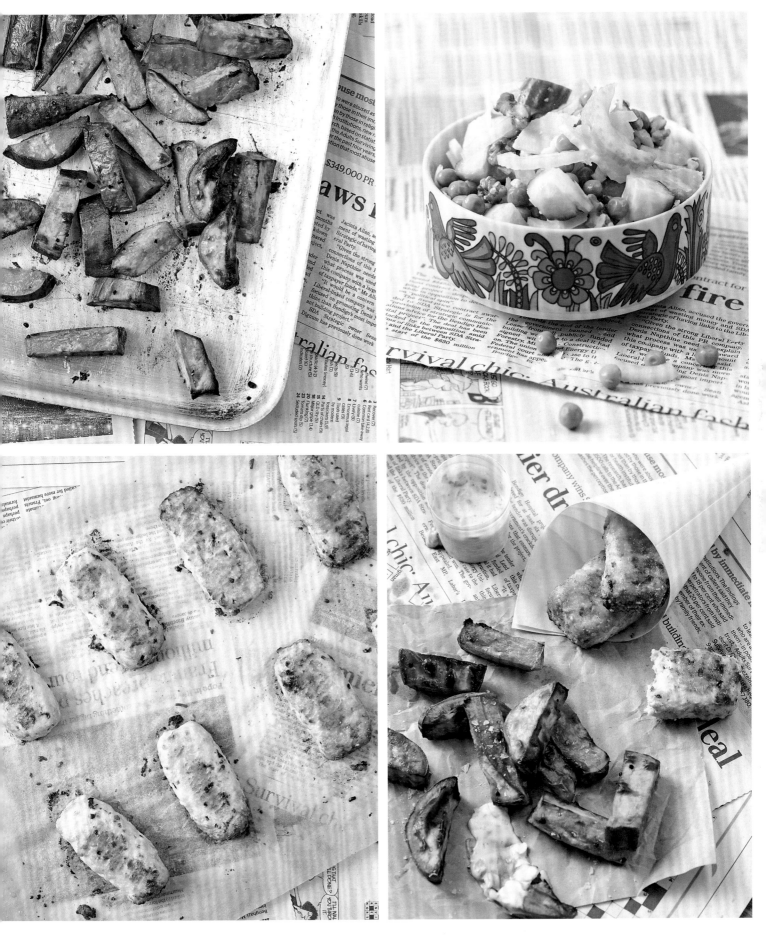

KFC *Kid-friendly chicken*

You won't want to touch the one with the secret herbs and spices after tasting this finger-lickin' version, made with secret (disguised) extra-dense nutrition. Soaking the chicken in buttermilk helps keep the meat juicy during baking. You can easily make your own buttermilk: mix ½ cup (125 ml) of full-fat milk with 2 tablespoons of lemon juice and set aside for 5 minutes.

Prepare the chicken by whisking the buttermilk with the mustard in a large glass bowl until well blended. Add the chicken and turn to coat, then cover and marinate in the fridge for at least 30 minutes and up to 8 hours.

Preheat the oven to 200°C (gas 6) and line a baking tray with baking paper. Throw the flour, baking powder, sesame seeds, paprika, garlic powder, salt and pepper into a medium zip-lock bag. Shake 1 or 2 pieces of marinated chicken at a time in the bag, until coated. Shake off excess flour and place the chicken on the prepared baking tray. Spray the chicken pieces lightly on both sides with olive oil spray if you like. Bake until golden brown and no longer pink in the centre, about 30 minutes for the thighs or 45 minutes for the drumsticks.

While the chicken is cooking, make the green mash by placing the potatoes in a saucepan of cold water over high heat. Bring to the boil, then reduce to a rolling simmer and cook for about 10 minutes, or until the potatoes are tender. Add the peas and broccoli, and cook for another 3 minutes, then drain and add the mint and oil or butter. Mix well, then mash the lot using a fork. Season with salt and pepper.

Prepare the slaw by combining the coleslaw, spring onion and mayo in a bowl.

To make the gravy, mix the hot Cauliflower Cream and cheese with a fork in a small bowl until the cheese has melted through.

Serve the KFC with the mash, gravy and slaw.

SOLO COOKERS: Tote drumsticks for lunch the next day and freeze any extra portions of cooked chicken for 2–3 months

DAIRY-FREE: For a dairy-free marinade, mix together 6 cups (1.5 litres) of water, 2 tablespoons of sea salt and 1 tablespoon of Dijon mustard. Add the chicken, cover with aluminium foil and marinate in the fridge for 4 hours. Drain and follow the recipe as normal.

½ cup (125 ml) buttermilk

1 tablespoon Dijon mustard

8 chicken drumsticks or chicken thighs

⅔ cup (75 g) plain flour, coconut or gluten-free plain flour

1 teaspoon baking powder

2 tablespoons sesame seeds

1½ teaspoons paprika

2 teaspoons garlic powder

1 teaspoon finely ground sea salt

1 teaspoon finely ground black pepper

olive oil cooking spray (optional)

MUSHY EXTRA GREEN PEAS

2 medium potatoes, peeled and cut into quarters

1 cup (150 g) frozen peas

2 cups (450 g) thawed Par-Cooked 'n' Frozen broccoli florets (see page 51)

5 mint leaves, finely chopped

2 tablespoons olive oil or butter

sea salt and freshly ground black pepper

SLAW

200 g undressed coleslaw mix or shredded red cabbage mixed with 1 carrot, cut into thin batons

4 spring onions or ½ small red onion, finely sliced

Whey-Good Mayo (see page 208)

CHEESY 'GRAVY'

½ quantity of Cauliflower Cream (see page 100)

⅓ cup (40 g) grated cheddar cheese

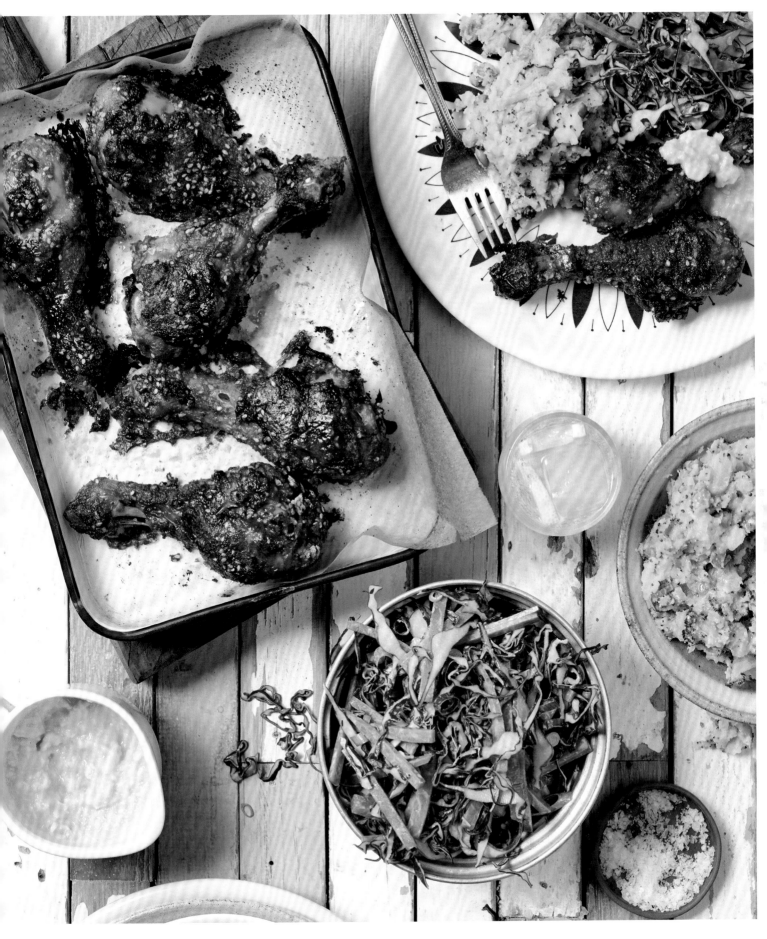

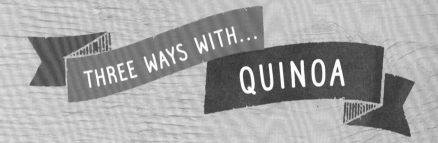

1. LEBANESE FALAFEL ROLLS

To make the quinoa falafel, use a food processor to blend the chickpeas with the harissa and coriander stalks until almost smooth. Transfer to a mixing bowl, then add the lemon zest and juice, quinoa, egg and coconut flour. Mix well to combine. Form into 12 patties using about 4 tablespoons of mixture for each one. Heat the olive oil in a frying pan over medium–high heat. Fry the falafel on each side until browned and crusty, in batches if needed.

Make the garlic sauce by mixing the yoghurt with the garlic and coriander leaves.

To serve, stuff each pitta pocket with 3 falafel, top with tabouleh and drizzle over the garlic sauce.

NOTE: How to prepare cooked quinoa. Rinse 1 cup (225 g) of quinoa well. Put it in a saucepan and pour in 500 ml water. Cover and bring to the boil, then reduce the heat and simmer, covered, for 15 minutes until all the water has been absorbed. Remove from the heat and let stand for 5 minutes, covered. Fluff with a fork. Makes 4 cups (540 g).

SUSTAINABILITY TIP: The remaining coriander leaves can be used in an Anti-Inflammatory Green Glowin' Skin Smoothie (see page 77) or made into stock cubes (see page 195).

VEGAN: Replace the egg in the falafel with 2 tablespoons chia seeds blended with some warm water.

V 8WP

SERVES **4** [MAKES 12 FALAFEL]

4 wholemeal pitta pockets or gluten-free mountain bread

QUINOA FALAFEL
2 × 400 g cans chickpeas, drained

1 tablespoon harissa paste or 2 tablespoons harissa powder

4 sprigs coriander, stalks chopped (reserve some of the leaves for the Garlic Sauce, below)

grated zest of 1 lemon

1 tablespoon lemon juice

1 cup (135 g) cooked quinoa (see note)

1 egg

¼ cup (25 g) coconut flour

2 tablespoons olive oil

GARLIC SAUCE
½ cup (125 ml) Greek-style full-fat organic plain yoghurt

2 teaspoons garlic powder or 3 cloves garlic, finely chopped

Red Pepper Tabouleh (see page 96), to serve

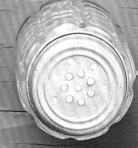

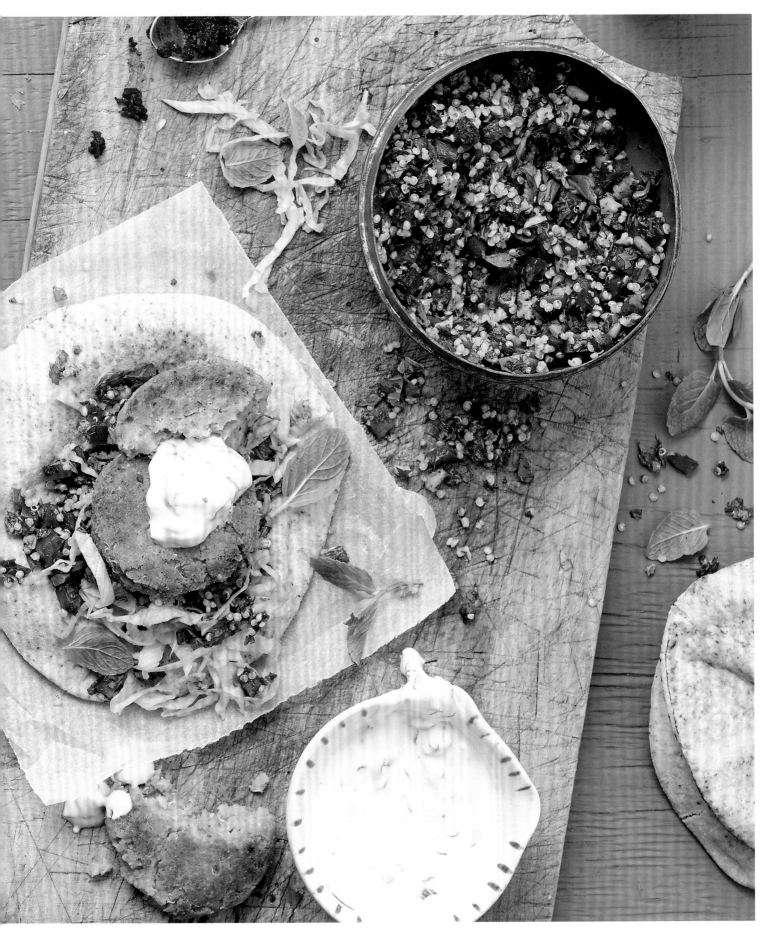

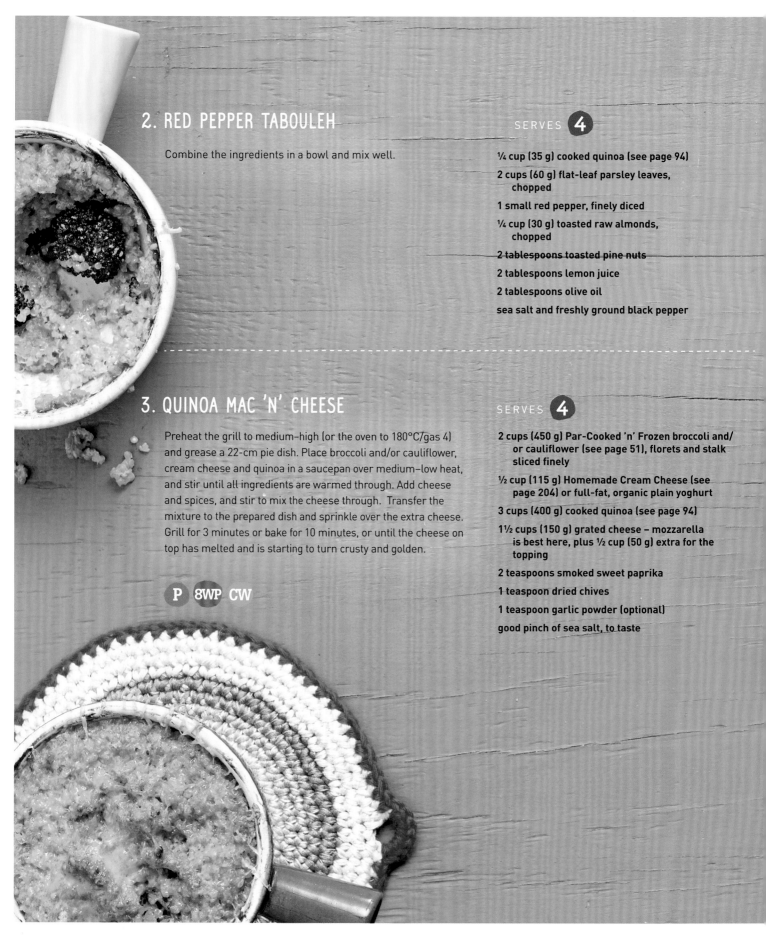

2. RED PEPPER TABOULEH

Combine the ingredients in a bowl and mix well.

SERVES **4**

¼ cup (35 g) cooked quinoa (see page 94)

2 cups (60 g) flat-leaf parsley leaves, chopped

1 small red pepper, finely diced

¼ cup (30 g) toasted raw almonds, chopped

2 tablespoons toasted pine nuts

2 tablespoons lemon juice

2 tablespoons olive oil

sea salt and freshly ground black pepper

3. QUINOA MAC 'N' CHEESE

Preheat the grill to medium–high (or the oven to 180°C/gas 4) and grease a 22-cm pie dish. Place broccoli and/or cauliflower, cream cheese and quinoa in a saucepan over medium–low heat, and stir until all ingredients are warmed through. Add cheese and spices, and stir to mix the cheese through. Transfer the mixture to the prepared dish and sprinkle over the extra cheese. Grill for 3 minutes or bake for 10 minutes, or until the cheese on top has melted and is starting to turn crusty and golden.

P **8WP** **CW**

SERVES **4**

2 cups (450 g) Par-Cooked 'n' Frozen broccoli and/or cauliflower (see page 51), florets and stalk sliced finely

½ cup (115 g) Homemade Cream Cheese (see page 204) or full-fat, organic plain yoghurt

3 cups (400 g) cooked quinoa (see page 94)

1½ cups (150 g) grated cheese – mozzarella is best here, plus ½ cup (50 g) extra for the topping

2 teaspoons smoked sweet paprika

1 teaspoon dried chives

1 teaspoon garlic powder (optional)

good pinch of sea salt, to taste

MIDDLE EASTERN MEATZA

A meatza? Yep, a meat-based pizza.

Preheat the oven to 200°C (gas 6) and line the base of a 23-cm pie dish or a spring-form cake tin with baking paper. In a large bowl, mix together the beef and spices. Spread the mince over the base of the prepared tin, pressing it down into the edges – the crust should be even all around and about 1 cm thick. Bake for 10–15 minutes or until the edges are beginning to brown. Remove from the oven and pat dry with kitchen paper, removing any juices from the sides if necessary.

Arrange the yoghurt, onion, pine nuts, asparagus and cheese on top. Return to the oven and bake for another 10 minutes or until the cheese has melted. Meanwhile, toss the rocket leaves with the olive oil and lemon juice. Remove the meatza from oven and arrange the dressed rocket on top to serve.

SOLO COOKERS: Before adding the rocket topping, divide into four and freeze extra portions individually for 2–3 months.

500 g lean organic beef mince

1 teaspoon smoked sweet paprika

2 teaspoons garlic powder

2 teaspoons ground cumin

1 teaspoon ground allspice

⅓ cup (75 ml) Greek-style full-fat organic plain yoghurt

1 small red onion, finely sliced

2 teaspoons pine nuts

1 bunch asparagus, trimmed

¼ cup (25 g) finely grated parmesan cheese

1 teaspoon chilli flakes (optional) or to taste

large handful of rocket leaves

½ tablespoon olive oil

squeeze of lemon juice

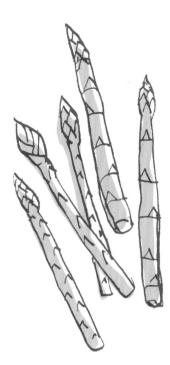

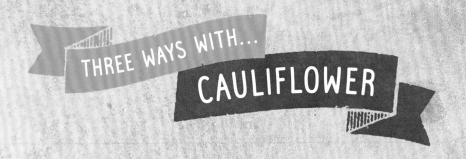

1. NOT SO NIÇOISE CAULIFLOWER PIZZA

Preheat the oven to 200°C (gas 6) and line a baking tray with baking paper. To make the crust, mix the cauliflower with the cheese and egg in a bowl, and season with salt and pepper. Using a wooden spoon or your hands, shape the mixture into 1 large pizza base or 4 small crusts. The bases should be about 1–1.5 cm thick. Bake for about 30–35 minutes, or until firm and golden, then remove from the oven.

To make the topping, mix the curry powder into the yoghurt and spread the mixture to the edges of the crust. Scatter with the tender stem broccoli, onion, capers, feta, olives, tuna and anchovies, then break the eggs in the middle. Bake for a further 8–10 minutes, or until the egg white is set. Finish with a sprinkle of salt and pepper on top.

SOLO COOKERS: Make the crust as per the recipe above, dividing the crust mixture into four individual crusts to cook. Freeze the extra bases. Defrost the crusts, top with one quarter of the topping amounts and grill instead of turning on the oven just for one serve.

FOURSOME FAMILIES: This recipe makes for a light meal and you can do a simple weekend lunch version with ham and cheese as your toppings. Extend it to a full meal by doubling the recipe and adding extra greens.

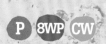

SERVES **4** [SMALL SERVINGS]

CRUST

1 medium-sized cauliflower, grated (by hand or in a food processer until rice-sized, but not pulverised) and cooked, well drained, cooled slightly

100 g goat's cheese or grated cheddar cheese

1 egg

sea salt and freshly ground black pepper

TOPPING

½ teaspoon curry powder

¼ cup (60 ml) Greek-style full-fat organic plain yoghurt

2 stalks broccolini (tender stem broccoli), sliced into 4 lengths

½ small red onion, finely sliced

2 teaspoons capers

½ cup (115 g) diced feta

¼ cup (40 g) small pitted olives

195 g can sustainably fished tuna in olive oil

4 anchovy fillets

2–3 eggs

sea salt and freshly ground black pepper

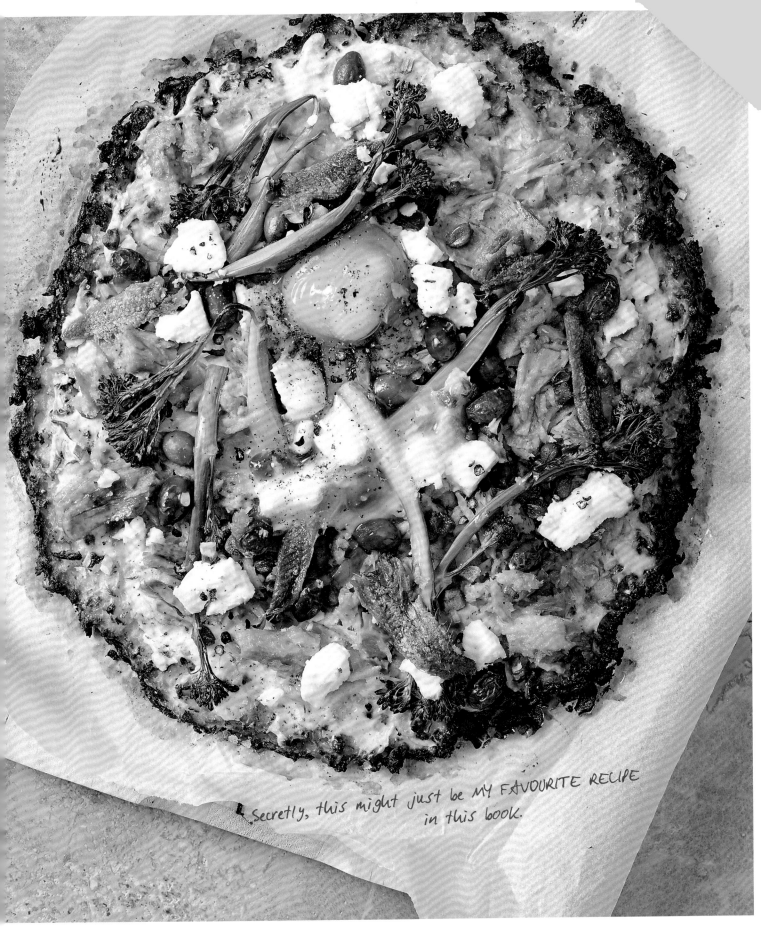

Secretly, this might just be MY FAVOURITE RECIPE
in this book.

CAULIFLOWER CREAM

SERVES 4

This cream makes for a less starchy and more densely nutritious substitute for mashed potato and can be served as a side with the slow-cooked dishes, and used to make a kid-adored Cheesy 'Gravy' (see page 92).

Place the cauliflower, cream and butter in a saucepan, season with salt, then cover and cook over low heat for 35 minutes. Blend until smooth using a stick blender or a potato masher.

½ cauliflower, broken into florets
½ cup (125 ml) cream
2 tablespoons butter
sea salt

 P **8WP** **CW**

---

3. CAULIFLOWER 'FRIED RICE'

SERVES 4

If I weren't flagging it right here, I bet you wouldn't notice this recipe is rice-free. I'm not averse to rice, I'm simply very pro adding as many extra vegetables to your day as possible.

Grate the cauliflower on the larger side of a cheese grater, or pulse in a food processor until it's rice-sized (but not pulverised). Wrap the riced cauliflower in a couple of paper towels and squeeze it to remove any excess moisture.

Heat ½ tablespoon of the oil in a frying pan over medium heat, then cook the eggs as a flat omelette. Remove from the pan and slice into strips using a knife or a pair of scissors and set aside. Heat the remaining oil in the same pan over medium heat and sauté the garlic. Add the carrot and peas and a splash of water to prevent sticking, and cook for 5 minutes. Add the spring onions, riced cauliflower and prawns, along with a generous splash of tamari or soy sauce and salt, to taste. Stir to combine and cook for a further 3–5 minutes.

1 small cauliflower
1½ tablespoons coconut oil or olive oil
4 eggs, lightly beaten
4 cloves garlic, finely chopped
2 carrots, diced
1 cup (150 g) frozen peas
6 spring onions, sliced
300 g cooked prawns, shelled
tamari or soy sauce, to taste
sea salt

SOLO COOKERS: Make the full quantity of cauliflower 'fried rice' and freeze three-quarters of it. Then adjust the remaining ingredients for 1 or 2 serves.

VEGAN: Use crumbled tofu instead of egg and sprinkle with sesame seeds or other seeds and/or nuts for extra protein.

BUYING PRAWNS: Ensure you buy local prawns only – those from Asian farms are a sustainability nightmare. Frozen or cooked prawns are fine to use, but if you plan on freezing some in bulk, buy only fresh, unfrozen ones (fish should only be frozen once).

P **V**

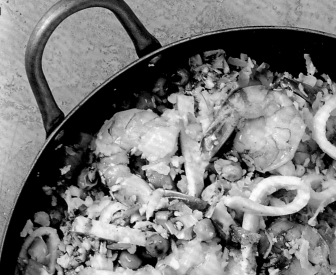

BAKED SATAY CHICKEN POPS

A spring roll with a baked-not-fried healthsome slant, these takeaway classics are a great way to use up leftover chicken and pumpkin. Perfect for kids' parties and sleepovers, too.

Preheat the oven to 180°C (gas 4) and line a baking tray with baking paper. Place all the ingredients except the spring roll wrappers, oil and dipping sauce in a bowl and mix well to combine. Working with 1 sheet at a time, place about 4 tablespoons of filling on the bottom third of each wrapper. Fold over the sides, then, working from the bottom end, roll up the wrapper and stuffing to form a lovely snug log. Place on the prepared tray and brush lightly with the olive oil. Bake for 15 minutes, turning halfway, or until the rolls are golden. Serve with vegetable sticks and the dipping sauce.

GLUTEN-FREE: Use rice paper rounds instead to make a 'raw' version. Soften rounds by soaking for about 1 minute each in a shallow dish filled with lukewarm water. Remove from dish and lay flat on a clean tea towel and follow the instructions as above, skipping the baking step.

2 cups (300 g) finely shredded cooked chicken (use leftovers from Crispy Roast Chook, see page 111)

1 cup (75 g) finely shredded lettuce

2 teaspoons ground coriander

1 teaspoon curry powder

½ cup (125 ml) Pumpkin Purée (see page 51)

handful of mint leaves

2 teaspoons sesame seeds

12 × 18-cm spring roll wrappers

olive oil, for greasing

vegetable sticks (carrots and celery – cut into batons – and mangetout), to serve

Satay Sauce or Deceptively Sweet Chilli Sauce (see page 207), for dipping

THAI FIX

Look out for this stamp if you are after 'sweet' Thai alternatives.

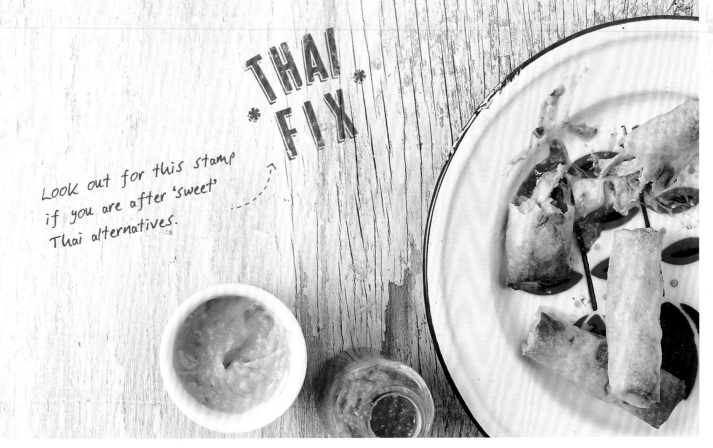

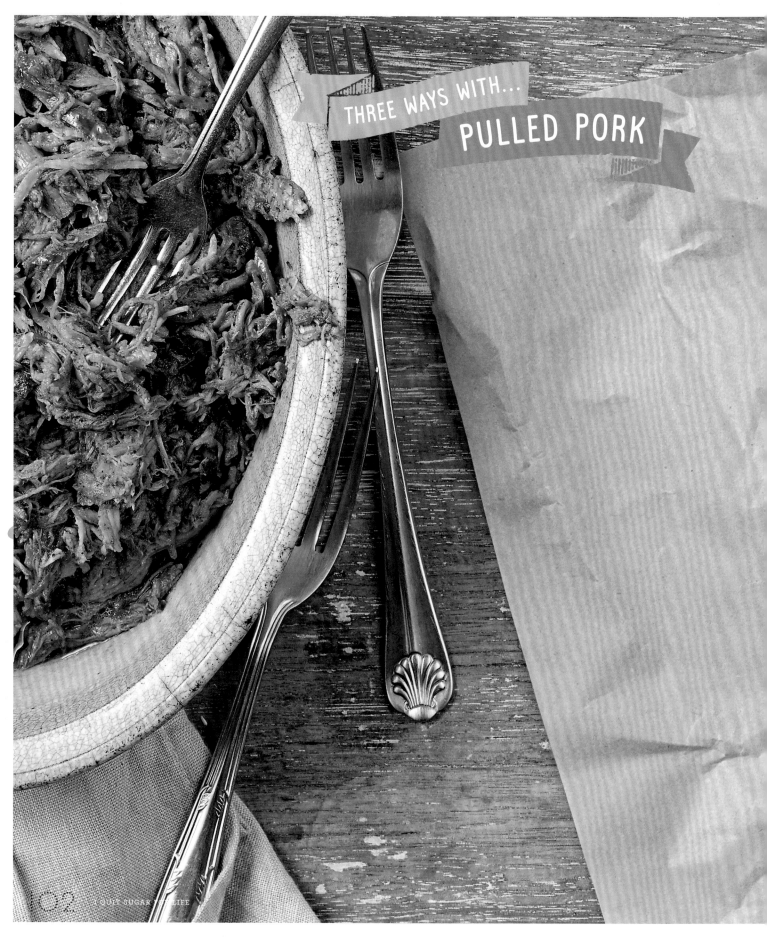

1. SLOW-COOKED BARBECUE PORK

SERVES **6**

Traditionally this dish is made using a lot of sugar and smoke. I developed this recipe to get around such impasses (most of us don't have a smokehouse in our backyards, right?). I rub the pork in fennel and salt instead of sugar and use 'smoked' sweet paprika to get the 'fumin'' taste. It's best to start making this the night before. Oh, and I make it to serve 6 so that families can also use the leftovers for sandwiches or wraps the next day, or to make the Banh Mi and tacos (see page 104).

Grind the fennel seeds and peppercorns using a mortar and pestle (or in a blender). Add the salt, paprika, cumin, allspice or cinnamon and chilli powder, and mix well. Rub the spice mixture over the pork, rubbing well into the fatty bits. Really get your fingers into the meat, massaging it all over. Leave covered in the fridge for at least 2 hours (for a stronger flavour I reckon you could leave it overnight).

Once you've 'cured' the meat, rub the oil into it and sear in a hot frying pan until brown all over (I don't usually brown my meat first when slow-cooking, but here it adds to the barbecue effect). Whack in an electric slow cooker and add the remaining ingredients. Cook on low for 8 hours or on high for 5 hours.

Take out the pork, place it in a dish and use a fork to 'pull the meat' into shreds. Put the shreds back into the slow cooker with the sauce and cook for another 20 minutes, uncovered, on high.

Serve 4 portions with the relish, greens and Cauliflower Cream.

SOLO COOKERS + FOURSOME FAMILIES: This will make 6 portions. Freeze any remaining meat in ½ cup (125 ml) portions in zip-lock bags and use to make the 'Pork Banh Mi' or taco recipes on the following page.

NOTE: The traditional cut for pork is the shoulder, which can be very large and won't fit into a standard (4.5-litre) electric slow cooker. Ask your butcher to cut off the bone-in end or use the neck (often called scotch or 'butt' in America). It's more expensive, but smaller.

P **8WP**

Ingredients

- 2 teaspoons fennel seeds
- 1½ teaspoons black peppercorns
- 3 teaspoons sea salt
- 3 teaspoons smoked sweet paprika (plain sweet paprika is fine, too)
- 1 teaspoon ground cumin
- 1 teaspoon ground allspice or cinnamon
- 2 teaspoons chilli powder
- 1–1.5 kg piece pork neck or pork shoulder (preferably bone in)
- 2 tablespoons olive oil or coconut oil
- 2 bay leaves
- ½ cup (125 ml) red wine or stock
- ⅓ cup (75 ml) apple cider vinegar
- ¼ × 440 g can whole peeled tomatoes, chopped, with some of the liquid
- 2 cloves garlic, finely chopped
- 2 tablespoons rice malt syrup
- Beetroot and Apple Relish (see page 199), steamed greens (see pages 128–9) and Cauliflower Cream (see page 100), to serve

CHEAT'S TRICK

Rub the meat in salt only and cook in ¾ cup (180 ml) of stock, then toss the shredded meat through 1 cup (240 ml) of my sugar-free Homemade BBQ Sauce (see page 206).

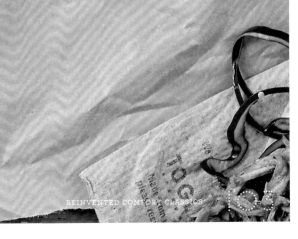

2. PORK BANH MI

These Vietnamese-style sandwiches are great vehicles for leftover pork.

In a small frying pan, heat the pork, adding a little water or stock if required. Spread one side of the bread roll with the mayo. Line with the cucumber and carrot. Fill the roll with the pulled pork, top with onion, coriander and lime juice. Serve immediately.

GLUTEN-FREE: use a gluten-free wrap instead of the roll.

1 portion Slow-Cooked Barbecue Pork (see page 103)

1 soft bread roll, cut in half lengthways

2 tablespoons Whey-Good Mayo (see page 208)

Fermented Cucumbers (see page 199), sliced or Cucumber Salad (see below)

1 carrot, cut into thin batons

2 spring onions or ¼ small red onion, finely sliced

4 tablespoons coriander leaves, chopped roughly

squeeze of lime juice

3. KOREAN PORK TACOS WITH CUCUMBER SALAD

About 2 hours before serving, make the cucumber salad: using a potato peeler (or mandolin), peel the cucumber into long thin strips. Place in a bowl and mix in the chilli, vinegar and salt. Set aside to 'pickle' in the fridge for 2 hours.

Meanwhile, combine the coleslaw, onion, coriander and mayo in another bowl and set aside. In a small frying pan, heat the pork, adding a little water if required. Place half of the pork mixture onto each tortilla, top each with coleslaw and serve with the cucumber salad.

100 g undressed coleslaw mix or shredded red cabbage mixed with 1 carrot, cut into thin batons

2 spring onions or ¼ small red onion, finely sliced

2 ½ tablespoons chopped coriander leaves

2 tablespoons Korean Mayo (see page 209)

1 portion Slow-Cooked Barbecue Pork (see page 103)

2 corn tortillas, warmed through, to serve

CUCUMBER SALAD

¼ cucumber

pinch of chilli flakes

1 tablespoon apple cider vinegar or rice vinegar

pinch of salt

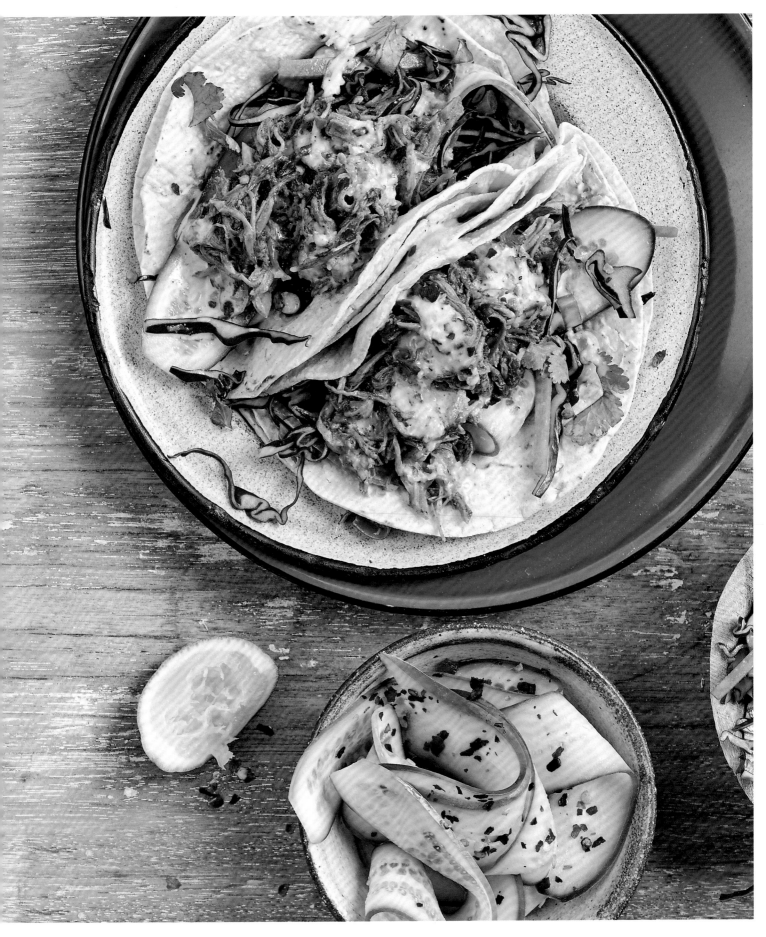

THAI RED CURRY 'BOLOGNAISE' WITH THAI-TALIAN SALAD

SERVES 4

This dish is double the healthy comfort – tomato-free bolognaise and a sweet Thai dish in one. It's made even more fun with a mock Mediterranean salad.

Heat the oil in a large saucepan over medium–high heat and add the onion and pepper. Cook for a minute or so, for the veggies to soften. Add the pork mince, five-spice and curry paste and, using a spoon or whisk, break the meat into smaller chunks and cook for another 5 minutes or so, until the mince is browned and cooked evenly.

Add the coconut cream to the pan and stir well, then reduce the heat to medium and simmer, uncovered, for 10 minutes. Add the peas and cook for a further 5 minutes, to warm through.

Cook the pasta according to the packet instructions, then drain and add to the mince. Combine the Thai-talian Salad ingredients in a bowl. Serve the pasta and sauce in bowls with the salad as a side.

PALEO AND GLUTEN-FREE: Use courgette ribbons instead of pasta. Use gluten-free pasta or courgette 'pasta'. Simply peel ½ large courgette per serve in long pasta-like strips using a potato peeler.

2 tablespoons olive oil

1 onion, chopped

1 small red pepper, sliced

500 g pork mince

1 teaspoon five-spice mix

4 tablespoons red curry paste

440 g can coconut cream

½ cup (75 g) frozen peas

200 g spaghetti

coriander leaves, roughly chopped, to serve

THAI-TALIAN SALAD

2 cucumbers, halved lengthways and sliced

12 cherry tomatoes, halved

1 cup (100 g) mangetout, thinly sliced

½ teaspoon chilli flakes

½ cup (20 g) coriander leaves, roughly chopped

2 tablespoons Take-Me-Anywhere Asian Dressing (see page 205)

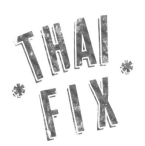

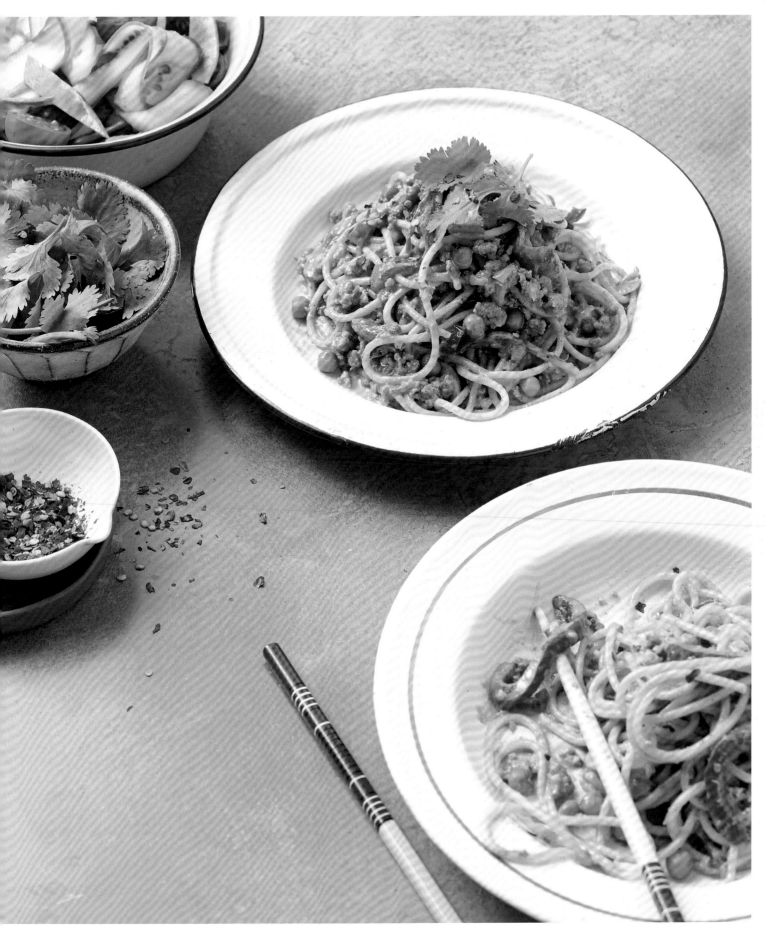

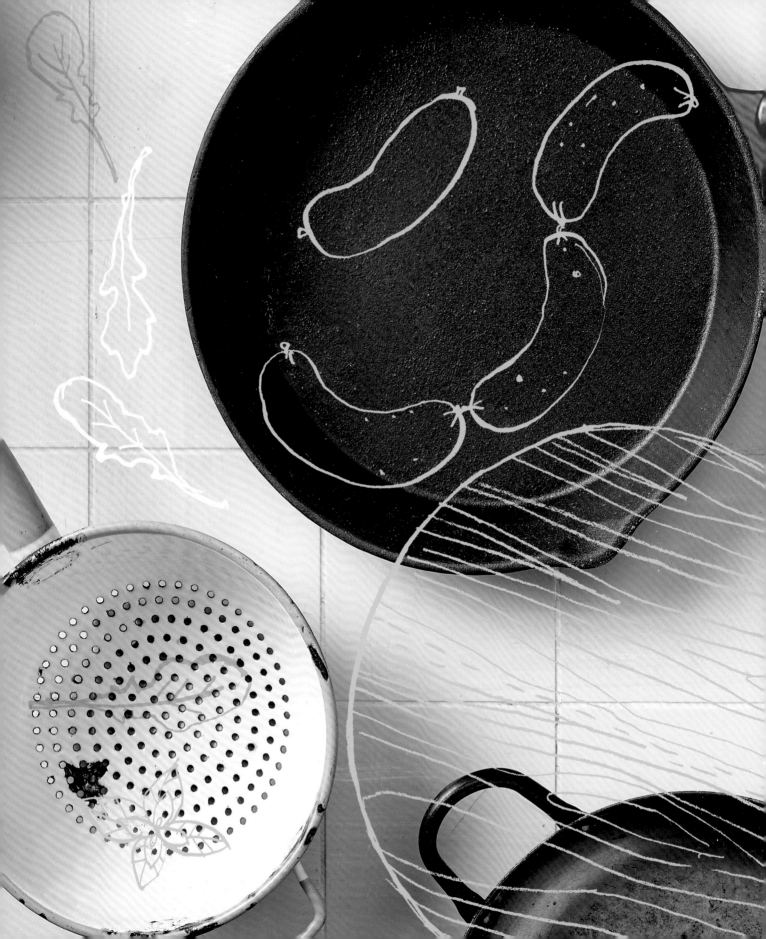

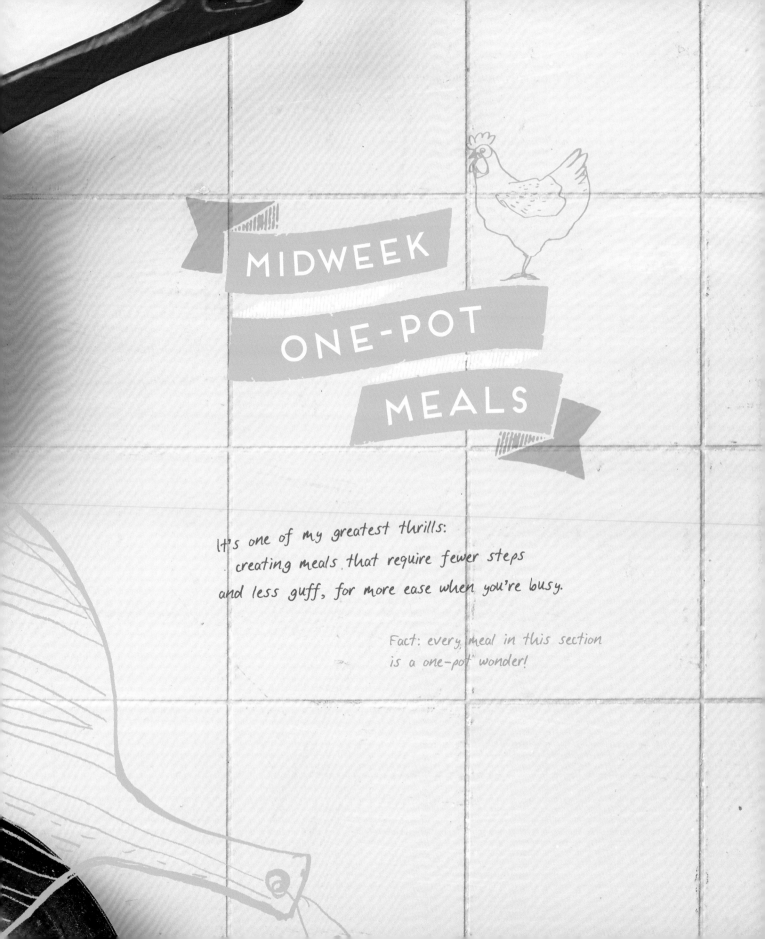

MIDWEEK ONE-POT MEALS

It's one of my greatest thrills:
  creating meals that require fewer steps
and less guff, for more ease when you're busy.

Fact: every meal in this section
  is a one-pot wonder!

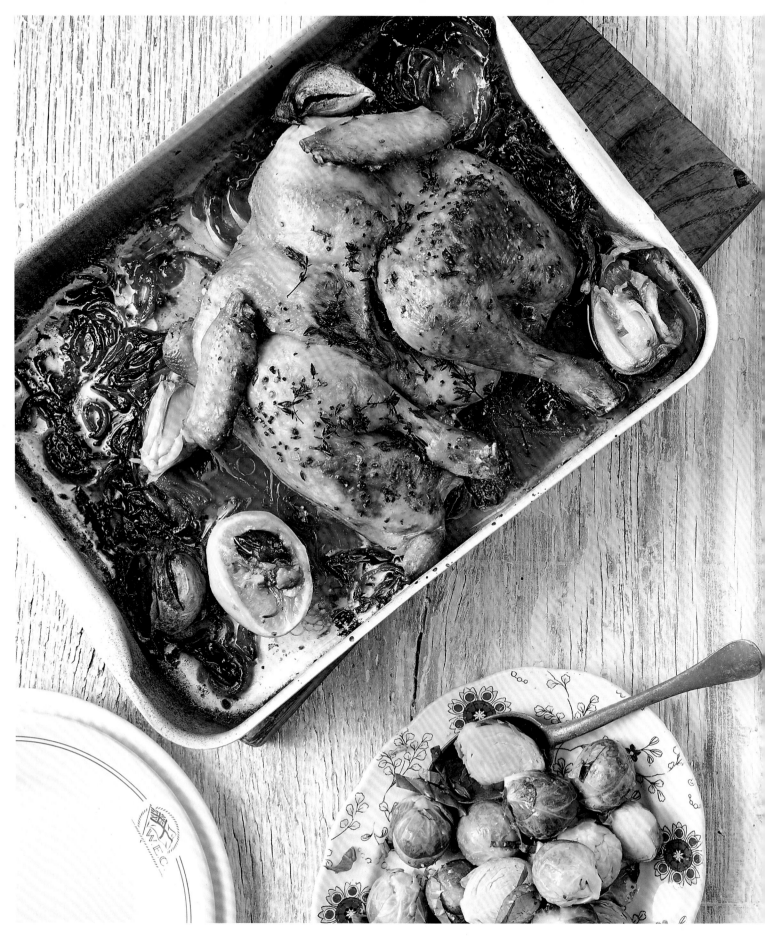

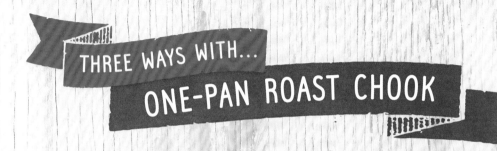

1. CRISPY ROAST CHOOK WITH SWEET POTATO CASSEROLE   SERVES 4-6

This roast chook recipe is one of my favourite mish-mash meals for it combines most of my eating principles in one tasty package: sustainability, economy and flow. It also combines the best of a number of flavour and cooking techniques, starting with cutting the whole chook in half, thus shortening the cooking time and not requiring constant turning, and, to my mind, making for a moister roast. Plonking things directly on top of the onion adds so much flavour, and stuffing butter under the skin ensures extra crispy skin. PS make sure you save your bones . . . you'll see why.

Preheat the oven to 200°C (gas 6). Toss the onion (except the ends) and garlic in a roasting pan. Using kitchen scissors, cut the chicken in half down either side of the backbone (the chunkier, bonier spine, not the smoother breast bone) and snap or cut the wings at the end joint and remove. Also cut off any chunky bits of fat.

Put the spine, wing ends and excess fat in a big stockpot with the onion end cuts and set aside to make some luscious Leftovers Chicken Stock (see page 191). If you don't have time to make stock immediately, just put the whole lot in a bag in the freezer, adding veggies, meat and herbs to the bag until you're ready to boil it all up.

Pat down the chicken, inside and out, with kitchen paper to ensure it's dry. Now, this is the fun bit: with the chicken breast-side up, using your fingers and working from the chicken's 'bottom' end, pull up the skin from the flesh and slide your fingers all the way up. Poke half the butter and some of the herbs up under the skin.

Squeeze the lemon halves over the chicken and rub the juice on both sides, retaining the lemon halves, then rub down with salt and pepper and the remaining herbs. Splay the chook and place in the roasting pan with the underside of the chicken on top of the onion and garlic, then place the squeezed lemon halves underneath and dot little chunks of the remaining butter over the top. Roast in the oven for 45 minutes, basting the chicken with the juices from the pan at 15 and 30 minutes.

To make the sweet potato casserole, lightly grease a small pie or baking dish using the oil, butter or ghee. Combine the sweet potato, almond milk, syrup, vanilla powder and salt, and pour into the baking dish. Toss the remaining ingredients in a small bowl, then sprinkle evenly over the top of the sweet potato mixture. Place in the oven with the chicken when the chicken has about 25 minutes to go.

1 onion, thinly sliced (keep the cut ends)

1 whole head garlic, cut into quarters

1 whole chicken, at room temperature

1 tablespoon butter

few sprigs of thyme or oregano

2 lemons, halved

sea salt and freshly ground black pepper

½ cup (125 ml) Leftovers Chicken Stock (see page 191), chicken stock, vermouth or dry white wine

SWEET POTATO CASSEROLE

coconut oil, butter or ghee, for greasing

3 cups (750 ml) Sweet Potato Purée (see Pumpkin Purée variation on page 51)

¼ cup (60 ml) almond milk

1 tablespoon rice malt syrup

1 teaspoon vanilla powder

pinch of sea salt

½ cup (60 g) chopped pecans (preferably activated; see page 204)

1 teaspoon ground cinnamon

½ teaspoon ground ginger

½ teaspoon ground allspice

steamed greens (see pages 128–9), to serve

[recipe continues next page]

[contd]

The chook will be ready when you poke a drumstick with a skewer and the juices run clear, not pink. When ready, remove the chook to an ovenproof serving dish, along with the garlic and lemon, then cover and leave in the still-warm oven (you can turn the oven off). Place the roasting pan over medium heat and deglaze with the stock, vermouth or wine: bring to the boil, scraping the onions and fatty bits off the bottom of the pan. Add a little more liquid if you like, then reduce. You can strain the sauce, but I prefer not to.

Cut the chicken into pieces and serve with the garlic, lemon and sauce, along with the sweet potato casserole and greens (Brussels sprouts work well).

SOLO COOKERS + FOURSOME FAMILIES: One large chook will make 6 portions. Once you've finished dinner, pull any remaining meat from the carcass and place in ½ cup (75 g) portions in zip-lock bags in the fridge or freezer. You can use these to make Roast Dinner Gratin (see opposite) or My Anti-Anxiety Soup (below).

SUSTAINABILITY TIP: Any leftover Sweet Potato Casserole can be reheated and eaten for breakfast or as a dessert with yoghurt or Whipped Coconut Cream (see page 72).

NOTE: Avoid roasting a frozen chook. They can be too watery. If you do use a frozen one, always thaw it in the fridge, uncovered, on some kitchen paper and pat it dry before cooking.

---

2. MY ANTI-ANXIETY SOUP

SERVES

Chicken soup is good for the soul: it fixes colds, it's the meal brought to the infirm and it's an incredible relaxant. How so? It works like this: the collagen released when you cook chicken bones (in particular) for hours feeds, repairs and calms the mucous lining of the small intestine. Our gut is our second brain and integral to our entire nervous system. Calm the gut, you calm your brain and body. Got it? This soup is embarrassingly simple and extraordinarily calming and nutritious. The swede gives it extra sweetness and earthiness.

Bring the broth to the boil, then reduce to a simmer and add the veggies. Cook for 1 minute, stir through the chicken and herbs and serve with black pepper to taste. Sip slowly.

NOTE: Swedes are a super-cheap and grounding root vegetable available in most supermarkets during winter. If you can't find one, use turnip or sweet potato.

1 cup (250 ml) Bone Broth made using chicken bones (see page 190)

½ courgette, cut into 1-cm dice

1 yellow squash, cut into 1-cm dice

¼ cup (40 g) diced (1 cm) swede

½ portion (4 tablespoons) shredded chicken (use leftovers from Crispy Roast Chook, see page 111 and above)

handful of chopped herbs (parsley is particularly good for a dose of minerals)

freshly ground black pepper

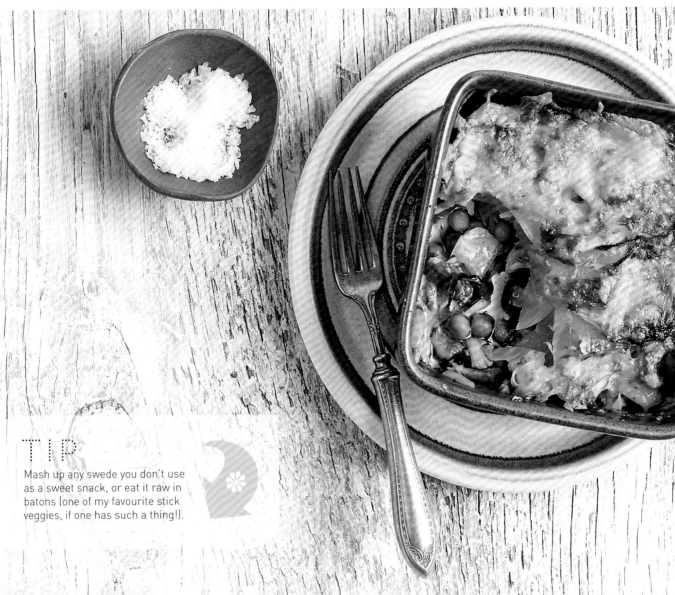

TIP

Mash up any swede you don't use as a sweet snack, or eat it raw in batons (one of my favourite stick veggies, if one has such a thing!).

3. ROAST DINNER GRATIN

Preheat the oven to 180°C (gas 4). Spread the shredded chicken over the bottom of a lightly greased ramekin or ovenproof bowl. Cook the peas and lightly steam the pumpkin, onion and cauliflower (if using a double steamer, place the peas on the bottom a few minutes ahead of putting the other vegetables on top). Layer the cooked vegetables over the chicken. Sprinkle the cheese over the lot. Bake for about 15 minutes or until the cheese has melted and browned. Serve with steamed greens.

SERVES **1**

1 portion shredded chicken (use leftovers from Crispy Roast Chook, see page 111)

½ cup (75 g) frozen peas

½ cup (75 g) finely wedged pumpkin

¼ onion, sliced

½ cup (115 g) defrosted and sliced or crumbled Par-Cooked 'n' Frozen cauliflower (see page 51)

⅓ cup (40 g) grated cheese (cheddar or parmesan)

steamed greens (see pages 128–9), to serve

GROUNDING ROOTS WINTER SOUP

In winter you have to get rooted. In the Ayurvedic tradition, the best way to stay well in winter is to pacify and warm the flighty, frenetic Vata energy that can build up over autumn by eating grounding foods. This soup is the perfect, calming anchor. The sweetness from the yoghurt and celeriac will further earth your flapping kite.

In a large, stainless-steel saucepan over very low heat, heat the 3 tablespoons of butter, oil or coconut oil and cook the leek and root vegetables gently and slowly, covered, for about 30 minutes. Add the garlic, herbs and spices and sweat a little more. Add the stock, season with salt and pepper, then bring to the boil. Reduce the heat and simmer, covered, for 20 minutes.

Meanwhile, heat the 1 teaspoon of butter, oil or coconut oil in a small frying pan over medium heat and cook the pancetta, turning once, until browned and crispy. Transfer to a plate lined with kitchen paper and allow to cool. Once cool, snap into shards.

Remove thyme and bay leaves from the soup and purée using a stick blender, or transfer to a blender and blitz in batches. Serve with a swirl of yoghurt and the pancetta shards scattered on top.

NOTE: I like to use white vegetables for this soup, but feel free to substitute carrot or sweet potato.

3 tablespoons butter, oil or coconut oil

2 leeks, chopped

5–6 cups (750–900 g) peeled and chopped root vegetables (e.g. 1 swede or turnip, 2 small parsnips, ½ celeriac)

3 cloves garlic, finely chopped

3 sprigs of thyme

2 bay leaves

¼ teaspoon cayenne pepper

½ teaspoon ground cumin

4 cups (1 litre) Leftovers Chicken Stock (see page 191)

sea salt and freshly ground black pepper

1 teaspoon butter, oil or coconut oil, for frying pancetta

6 slices pancetta

½ cup (125 ml) full-fat organic plain yoghurt

GREEK LONGEVITY SOUFIKO

SERVES 4

Consider this a lesson from the Ikarians in eating olive oil correctly like the Ikarians do. The Ikarians don't eat moderate amounts of olive oil, they eat lashings of it. Embrace their secret and use more than you're used to in this dish. Soufiko is a classic Ikarian dish served at almost every meal. It's basically fresh vegetables slow-cooked in oil.

The vegetables I've used here are best suited to summer. If something here isn't in season, use beans – flat or string – some okra, corn cobs, and so on, or up the amounts of the other vegetables. I personally like it best with just courgettes.

Layer the vegetables in a large frying pan with a heavy base and a lid, or a very shallow saucepan, in the order listed (i.e. the longest-to-cook vegetables on the bottom), seasoning with salt and pouring the olive oil over the top at the end. Cook over low heat, covered, for 20–30 minutes. Sprinkle oregano over the top and drizzle over extra olive oil to serve. Eat hot or cold with bread or Sardines 'n' Roots or yoghurt . . . and more oil!

1 large aubergine, cut into 2-cm pieces

2 onions, cut in half then sliced

2 cloves garlic, chopped

2 peppers (red or green or both), cut into 2-cm pieces

2 courgettes, cut into 2-cm pieces

2 tomatoes, cut into 2-cm pieces

2 teaspoons sea salt

½ cup (125 ml) olive oil, plus extra to serve

2 teaspoons good-quality dried oregano

full-fat organic plain yoghurt, to serve

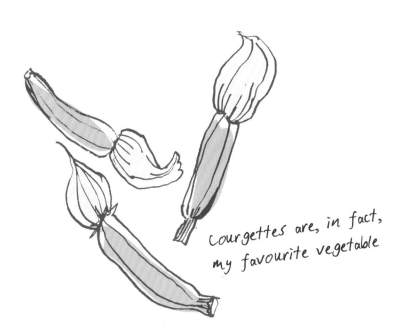

courgettes are, in fact, my favourite vegetable

ONE-PAN SARDINES 'N' ROOTS

SERVES 1

Sardines are the best fish. Period. They're super high in DHA, their edible bones are brimful of minerals, they are low in mercury and the most sustainable option at the fishmonger. They're currently not overfished, there's little or no by-catch and you can eat the whole thing. And they're dirt-cheap. PS Studies show oven-baking is the best way to preserve sardines' healthy oils.

You can buy sardines whole and fillet them yourself by cutting from just beneath the head down the belly and removing the gills and insides. Wash under running water and rub to remove blood and scales. Pat dry. (I personally eat the heads and tails . . . the best bit, ask any Italian.) Squeamish? Get the fishmonger to do it for you so you start with butterflied fillets.

Preheat the oven to 200ºC (gas 6). Arrange the root vegetables in an even layer on a greased baking dish or tray, season and drizzle with half the olive oil and bake for 20–25 minutes.

Place the sardines over and scatter the onion, garlic, herbs, chilli, plenty of pepper and salt and the lemon wedges around. Squeeze the juice of the reserved lemon over and the rest of the oil. Return to the oven and roast for 10 more minutes until the sardines are just cooked.

If you're cooking extra sardines, set these next to your roots, or place on another lightly greased tray, insides facing up, sprinkle with extra herbs, chilli flakes, pepper and salt and oil and cook at the same time (also for 10 minutes).

SOLO COOKERS + FOURSOME FAMILIES: This recipe is a one-pan-wonder-for-one, easily expandable to serve 4 or more. I recommend solo cookers cook up a bunch and then set aside to eat as below.

- 1–2 cups (150–300 g) sliced pumpkin, potato or sweet potato, skin on
- 1 tablespoon olive oil
- 4 sardines (16 if you're going to save some for the variations below. You can use tinned sardines for these recipes if you like)
- ¼ small red onion, thinly sliced
- 2 cloves garlic, smashed but skin on
- couple of sprigs of thyme or oregano or rosemary, chopped
- pinch of chilli flakes
- 1 lemon (½ cut into wedges, ½ reserved)
- sea salt and freshly ground black pepper (to taste, but be generous)

New York Variations:

During my recent visits to New York, I noticed sardines were quite de rigueur. Here are a few NYC-inspired recipes.

1. 'BLOODY MARY' TOASTIES

Crush 2 sardines with a dash of Homemade Tomato Sauce (see page 206), Tabasco and Worcestershire sauces, lemon juice (and a splash of vodka). Spread on toast.

2. PRUNE SARDINES ON BISCUITS

(Prune's a famous Manhattan brunch joint and they serve a version of this at their bar.) Mash 2 sardines with 1 teaspoon each of mustard and mayo and serve with a hearty cracker.

3. CHOPPED 'SHARP' SALAD WITH SARDINES

Simply serve a few sardines crumbled over a plate of chopped vegetables and herbs with a bit of tang (watercress, rocket, radish, fennel and red onion). Drizzle with oil and throw on some avocado for extra measure.

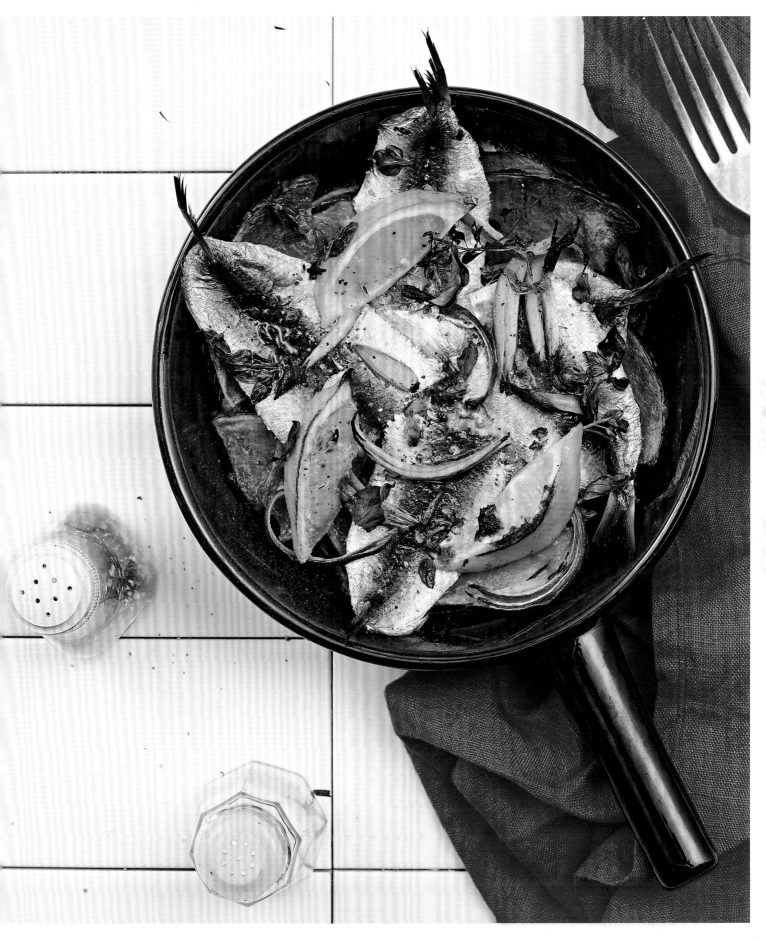

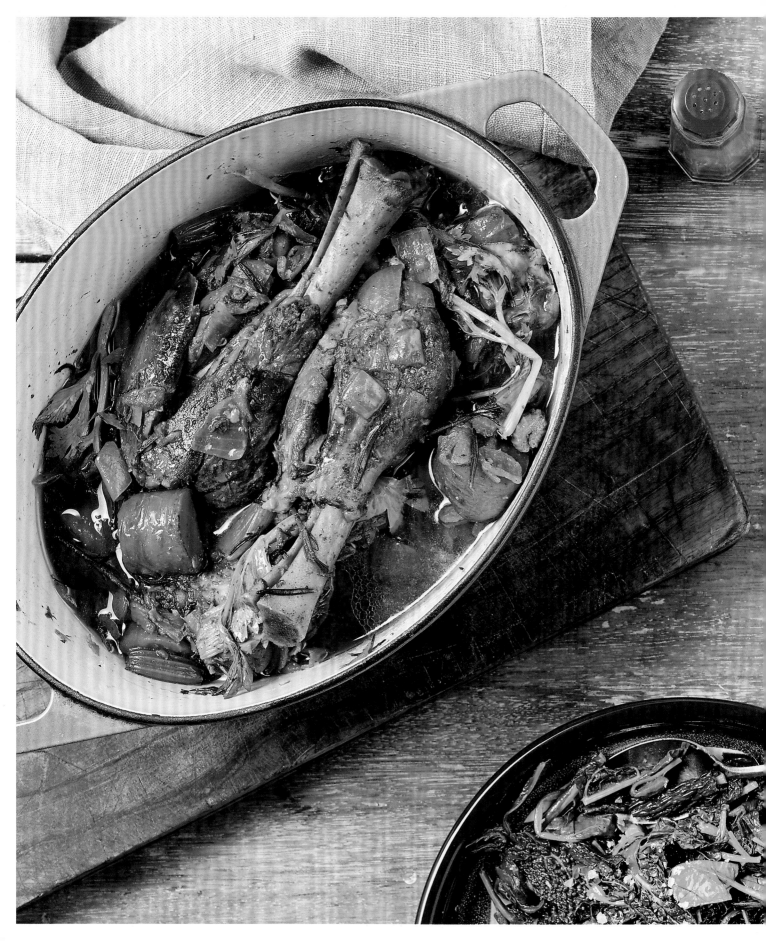

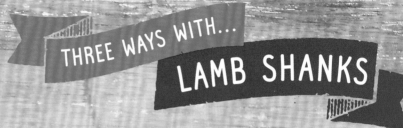

THREE WAYS WITH...
LAMB SHANKS

1. LEMON AND CINNAMON LAMB SHANKS WITH GREMOLATA

SERVES **6**

Between you and me, I find some shanks rather large and can often 'extend' 4 shanks to serve 6 by taking the meat off the bone, shredding it and returning it to the sauce before serving. Of course, I ensure I save any marrow from the bones – the best bit!

Throw the onion, carrot and celery (not the leaves) into a slow cooker. Arrange the shanks on top, then place the remaining ingredients (except the celery leaves, greens and cauliflower) over the lot. Stir a little (but don't worry about mixing completely). Put on the lid and cook for 4 hours on high or 8 hours on low.

Meanwhile, make the gremolata by combining all the ingredients in a jar and shaking. Serve one shank per person, with plenty of the sauce mixture, greens and Cauliflower Cream.

SOLO COOKERS + FOURSOME FAMILIES: Freeze any remaining meat in half cup (75 g) portions in zip-lock bags and use to make the Shanky Shepherd's Pie or Lamb Shank One-Pot Pasta recipes on the following pages. Also freeze the remaining sauce in 1-cup (250 ml) portions.

TIP

Freeze any leftover gremolata in an ice-cube tray. Pop out to use in soups, pastas or on toast.

1 onion, chopped

2 small carrots, cut into 2-cm chunks

2 celery stalks, cut into 2-cm chunks, reserving the leaves for the gremolata

4 lamb shanks (about 1 kg in total)

2 cloves garlic, crushed

½ cup (125 ml) Bone Broth (see page 190) or Leftovers Chicken Stock (see page 191), or water with good-quality stock powder or paste

½ cup (125 ml) red wine (or white wine or just a dash of apple cider vinegar)

1 bay leaf

4 sprigs of thyme or rosemary (or a good sprinkle of dried thyme)

½ teaspoon granulated stevia (optional)

1 tablespoon chopped preserved lemon, or grated zest and juice of 1 lemon

1 teaspoon ground cinnamon

steamed greens (see pages 128–9) and Cauliflower Cream (see page 100), to serve

LEMONY GREMOLATA

1 bunch flat-leaf parsley, very finely chopped

6–8 cloves garlic, very finely chopped

grated zest and juice of 2 lemons or 2 tablespoons chopped preserved lemon

4 tablespoons extra-virgin olive oil

1 teaspoon sea salt

chopped celery leaves, reserved from shanks (see above)

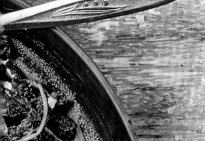

P 8WP-CW

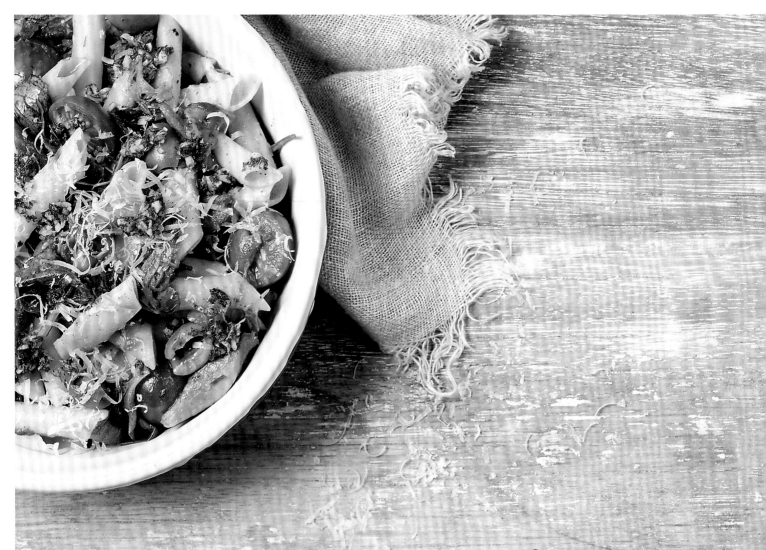

2. LAMB SHANK ONE-POT PASTA

Pour the liquid into a large stockpot and bring to the boil over high heat. Add the pasta and cook for about 5 minutes, then add the shredded lamb and olives, and stir through. Cook for a further 2 minutes for the meat to warm up and the pasta to cook through. Add the cherry tomatoes, baby spinach, cinnamon and pepper. Mix through and serve with a good grating of parmesan and the gremolata.

P **8WP**

SERVES **1**

½ cup (125 ml) lamb shank braising liquid

¾ cup (180 ml) water

100 g penne

1 portion leftover shank meat (see page 119), shredded

¼ cup (40 g) large pitted green olives, (feta-stuffed olives are great for this)

4 cherry tomatoes, halved (optional)

1 cup (30 g) baby spinach

ground cinnamon, to taste

freshly ground black pepper

parmesan cheese, to serve

leftover Lemony Gremolata (see page 119), to serve

3. SHANKY SHEPHERD'S PIE

Preheat the oven to 200°C (gas 6) and lightly grease a small pie dish or ramekin. Heat the oil, butter or ghee in a small saucepan and sauté the carrot and onion with the cumin until soft. Add the shredded meat and liquid or stock and simmer for 2–3 minutes. Spoon into the prepared pie dish or ramekin and spread the Sweet Potato Purée over the top. Dot with the butter and bake for about 25 minutes, or until golden.

FOURSOME FAMILIES: This recipe is easy to quadruple. You can also add a 440 g can brown lentils if you want to bulk it out further.

SERVES 1

1 teaspoon coconut oil, butter or ghee

1 small carrot, finely diced

½ onion, finely diced

¼ teaspoon ground cumin

1 portion leftover shank meat, shredded

2 tablespoons lamb shank braising liquid or any stock, or water with good-quality stock powder or paste

½ cup (125 ml) Sweet Potato Purée (see Pumpkin Purée variation on page 51)

1 tablespoon butter

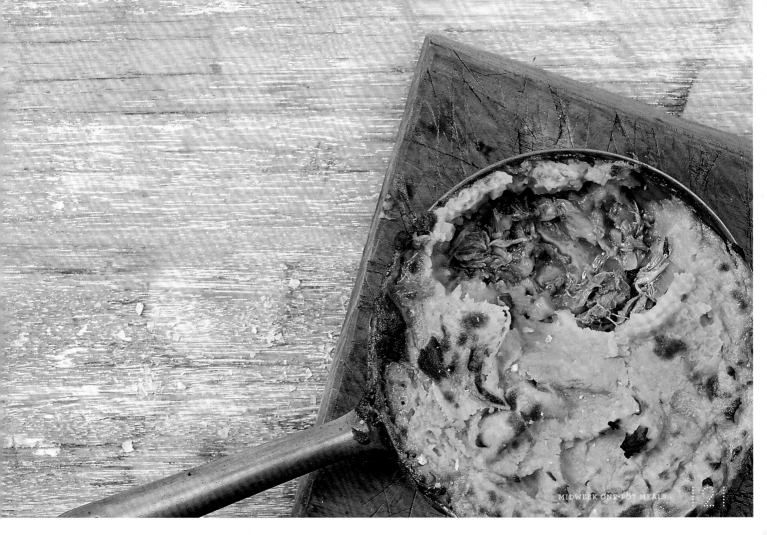

VIETNAMESE CHICKEN CURRY

The meal that made me cry!

OK, so when I'm asked to cite my favourite food experience, this is the one I share. I first ate cari ga on a mountain-bike trip with my brother Pete in Vietnam. We'd been riding for 9 hours through a desert and up one of the highest mountains in the country. Plus, I had food poisoning. By the time we arrived, I was deadset delirious. Pete found us a hole-in-the-wall place steaming with a cauldron of this Vietnamese version of chicken curry. At the first spoonful, I cried from the life-giving pleasure it injected into me and ordered another two serves. I keep a picture of it above my desk as a big reminder of the worth of getting over a mountain. Cari ga is traditionally made with potato and served with a chunk of baguette, but I've substituted sweet potato.

Place the chicken, chopped lemongrass, garlic, ginger, fish sauce and half the curry powder or paste in a bowl (it's best to use the ceramic insert from your electric slow cooker) and toss to combine. Cover and refrigerate for at least 1 hour to marinate. (You could even leave it overnight. I do.)

Transfer the mixture to the slow cooker (if you've marinated the chicken in the insert, simply replace the insert). Mix the rest of the curry powder or paste with a little of the stock, and add to the slow cooker along with the vegetables, the rest of the stock, the coconut milk, stevia, lemongrass ends and bay leaves. Stir to combine and cook on low for 7–8 hours or high for 3–4 hours.

If you like a thicker curry (I do), 20 minutes before serving, remove 4 tablespoons of the liquid from the slow cooker and whisk in the arrowroot, cornflour or chia bran to form a slurry, then pour back into the curry and stir through. Replace the lid, turn the slow cooker to high and cook for another 20 minutes.

Garnish with spring onions and serve with roti, mountain bread, poppadoms or a baguette.

- **700 g chicken thighs or chicken pieces, skin on and bone in**
- **1 stalk lemongrass, finely chopped, green ends reserved (or 1 tablespoon bought chopped lemongrass)**
- **2 cloves garlic, finely chopped**
- **3-cm knob of fresh ginger, finely chopped (or 1 tablespoon bought chopped ginger)**
- **2 tablespoons fish sauce**
- **5 tablespoons yellow curry powder or Massaman curry paste**
- **1 cup (250 ml) Leftovers Chicken Stock (see page 191)**
- **2 medium sweet potatoes, cut into 2.5-cm chunks**
- **1 large carrot, cut into 2.5-cm chunks**
- **1 onion, cut into 2.5-cm chunks**
- **400 ml can coconut milk**
- **½ teaspoon granulated stevia (optional)**
- **2 bay leaves**
- **2 tablespoons arrowroot, cornflour or chia bran (optional)**
- **2 spring onions, chopped**
- **roti, mountain bread, poppadoms or a baguette, to serve**

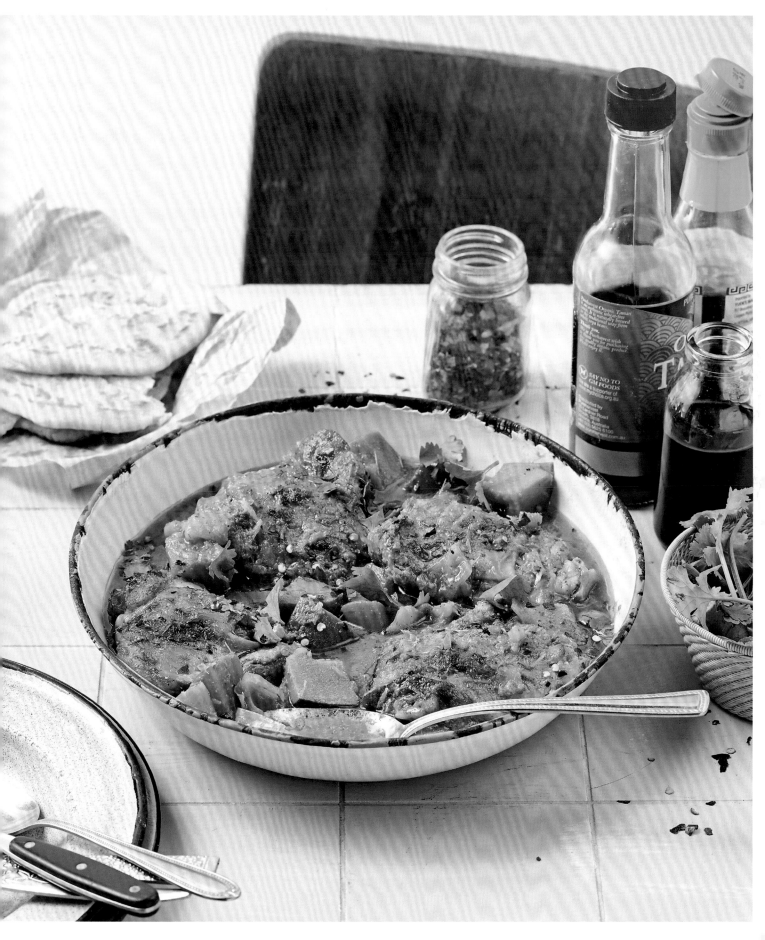

'ONE-POT-WONDER' SWEET CHILLI JAM AND CASHEW FISH

SERVES 4

Preheat the oven to 180°C (gas 4). Arrange broccolini (tender stem broccoli), basil and cashews in a large ovenproof dish. Top with the fish pieces and drizzle with sweet chilli sauce. Bake for about 15 minutes, or until the fish is cooked through. Serve garnished with the extra basil leaves.

Bulk-out Variation:

A clever way to bulk out this recipe for hungry families is to add rice. Place ½ cup (100 g) rice and 1½ cups (350 ml) water in a large ovenproof frying pan or a cast-iron skillet that will fit in the oven, cover with a lid or foil and bring to the boil over high heat, then reduce the heat to medium and simmer for 10 minutes – most of the water should be gone and the rice should be tender but still a little undercooked. Remove pan from heat. Follow the recipe as above, using the pan or skillet containing the rice base.

2 bunches broccolini (tender stem broccoli)

small handful of basil leaves, plus extra to serve

½ cup (75 g) cashews

600 g skinless whiting fillets, cut into even portions

½ cup (120 ml) Deceptively Sweet Chilli Sauce (see page 207)

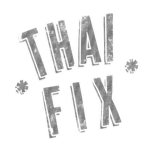

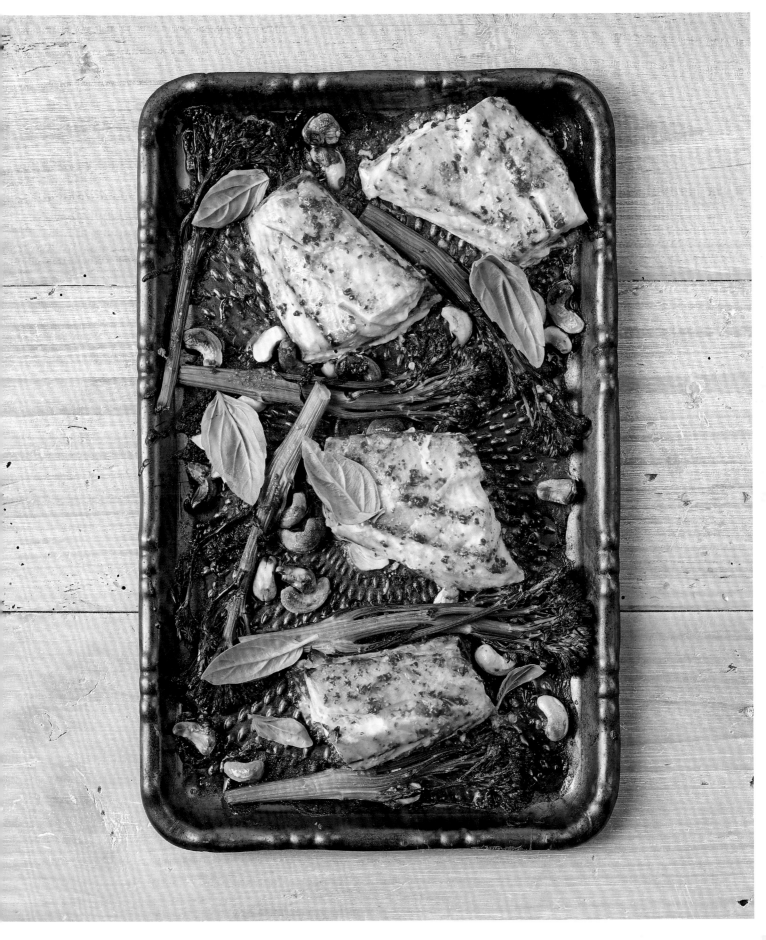

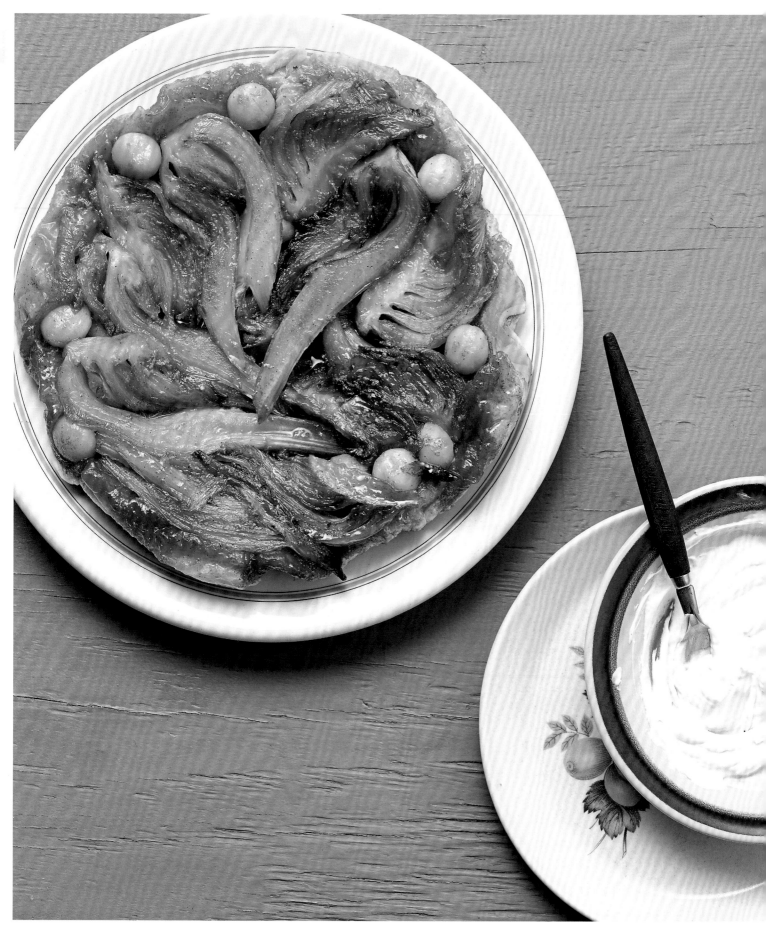

FENNEL TARTE TATIN

Travelling in Southern Europe, I've come across a lot of different ways to fix a fennel. When in season (during autumn), you should buy up these sweet-satiating, stomach-settling and inflammation-busting bulbs and make both versions of this twist on the French dessert classic. The sweet version is great for afternoon tea, the savoury for a weekend lunch.

Preheat the oven to 200°C (gas 6). In a large ovenproof frying pan, heat the oil over medium–high heat. Add the fennel wedges and cook for 4 minutes on each side or until golden and caramelised. Drizzle over the syrup and milk, and cook for another minute for the syrup to thicken. Arrange the fennel in a pattern in the pan. Add the macadamia nuts and sprinkle the lot with the cinnamon. Remove from the heat and cover with the puff pastry cut to fit. Pop in the oven and cook for 15–20 minutes or until the pastry is puffed and golden. To serve, gently dislodge the edges of the pastry from the pan using a fork or knife. Place a large plate upside down on top of the pan and flip the whole thing over. You may need to reshuffle a couple of the fennel wedges. Serve warm on its own or with a spoonful of yoghurt, cream or Whipped Coconut Cream.

Savoury Variation:
A CHEESY VERSION

Make as for the sweet tarte tatin, but replace the cinnamon with ½ tablespoon of thyme leaves and, instead of the Whipped Coconut Cream, top the cooked tarte with 125 g of soft goat's cheese, crumbled, and freshly ground black pepper to taste.

1 tablespoon coconut oil

2 medium bulbs fennel, trimmed and cut into wedges

⅓ cup (75 ml) rice malt syrup

2 tablespoons full-fat milk (or any other kind of milk)

½ (115 g) cup macadamia nuts

1 teaspoon ground cinnamon

1 sheet puff pastry or gluten-free puff pastry, thawed

full-fat organic plain yoghurt, cream or Whipped Coconut Cream (see page 72), to serve (optional)

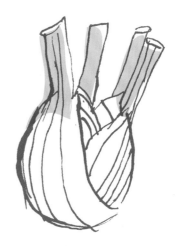

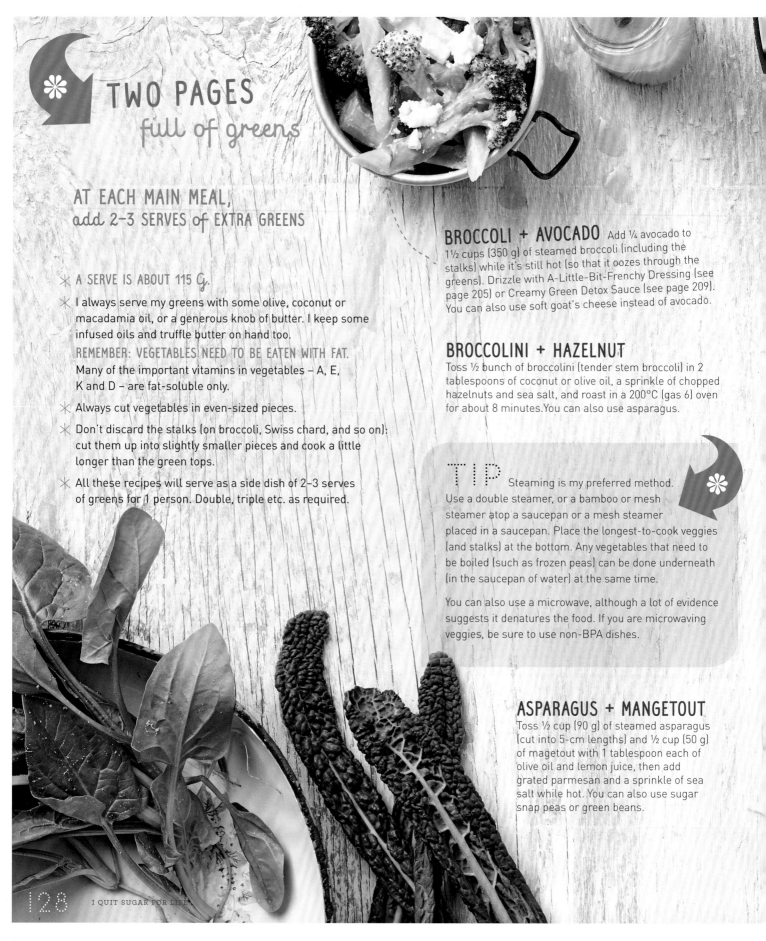

TWO PAGES
full of greens

AT EACH MAIN MEAL,
add 2–3 SERVES of EXTRA GREENS

✳ A SERVE IS ABOUT 115 G.

✳ I always serve my greens with some olive, coconut or macadamia oil, or a generous knob of butter. I keep some infused oils and truffle butter on hand too.
REMEMBER: VEGETABLES NEED TO BE EATEN WITH FAT.
Many of the important vitamins in vegetables – A, E, K and D – are fat-soluble only.

✳ Always cut vegetables in even-sized pieces.

✳ Don't discard the stalks (on broccoli, Swiss chard, and so on): cut them up into slightly smaller pieces and cook a little longer than the green tops.

✳ All these recipes will serve as a side dish of 2–3 serves of greens for 1 person. Double, triple etc. as required.

BROCCOLI + AVOCADO
Add ¼ avocado to 1½ cups (350 g) of steamed broccoli (including the stalks) while it's still hot (so that it oozes through the greens). Drizzle with A-Little-Bit-Frenchy Dressing (see page 205) or Creamy Green Detox Sauce (see page 209). You can also use soft goat's cheese instead of avocado.

BROCCOLINI + HAZELNUT
Toss ½ bunch of broccolini (tender stem broccoli) in 2 tablespoons of coconut or olive oil, a sprinkle of chopped hazelnuts and sea salt, and roast in a 200°C (gas 6) oven for about 8 minutes.You can also use asparagus.

TIP
Steaming is my preferred method. Use a double steamer, or a bamboo or mesh steamer atop a saucepan or a mesh steamer placed in a saucepan. Place the longest-to-cook veggies (and stalks) at the bottom. Any vegetables that need to be boiled (such as frozen peas) can be done underneath (in the saucepan of water) at the same time.

You can also use a microwave, although a lot of evidence suggests it denatures the food. If you are microwaving veggies, be sure to use non-BPA dishes.

ASPARAGUS + MANGETOUT
Toss ½ cup (90 g) of steamed asparagus (cut into 5-cm lengths) and ½ cup (50 g) of magetout with 1 tablespoon each of olive oil and lemon juice, then add grated parmesan and a sprinkle of sea salt while hot. You can also use sugar snap peas or green beans.

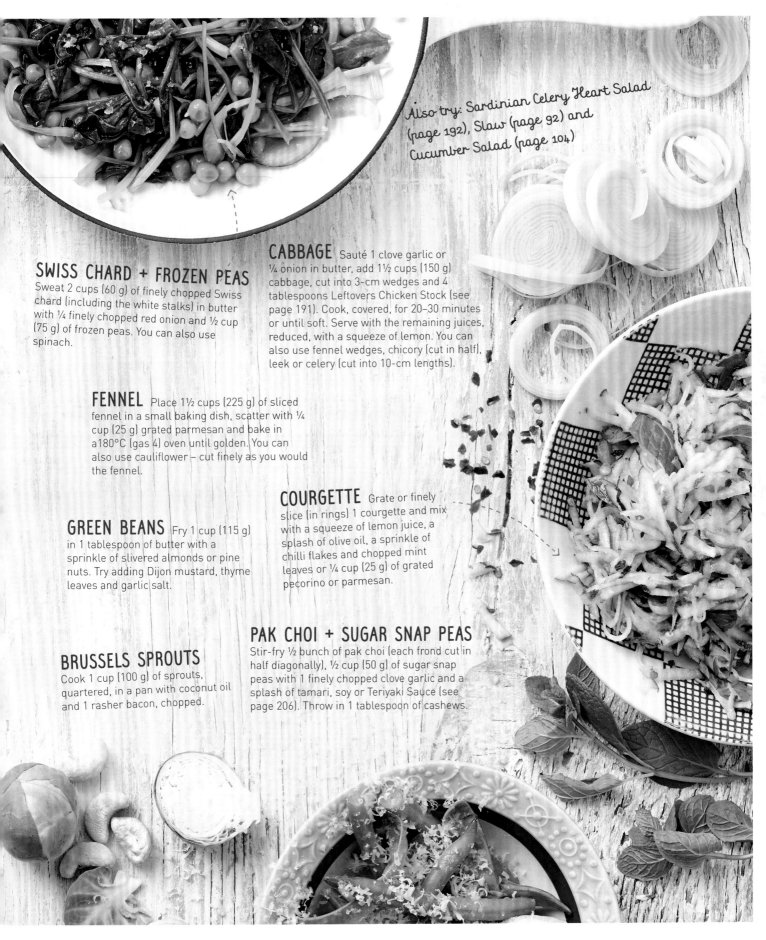

Also try: Sardinian Celery Heart Salad (page 192), Slaw (page 92) and Cucumber Salad (page 104)

SWISS CHARD + FROZEN PEAS

Sweat 2 cups (60 g) of finely chopped Swiss chard (including the white stalks) in butter with ¼ finely chopped red onion and ½ cup (75 g) of frozen peas. You can also use spinach.

FENNEL

Place 1½ cups (225 g) of sliced fennel in a small baking dish, scatter with ¼ cup (25 g) grated parmesan and bake in a180°C (gas 4) oven until golden. You can also use cauliflower – cut finely as you would the fennel.

GREEN BEANS

Fry 1 cup (115 g) in 1 tablespoon of butter with a sprinkle of slivered almonds or pine nuts. Try adding Dijon mustard, thyme leaves and garlic salt.

BRUSSELS SPROUTS

Cook 1 cup (100 g) of sprouts, quartered, in a pan with coconut oil and 1 rasher bacon, chopped.

CABBAGE

Sauté 1 clove garlic or ¼ onion in butter, add 1½ cups (150 g) cabbage, cut into 3-cm wedges and 4 tablespoons Leftovers Chicken Stock (see page 191). Cook, covered, for 20–30 minutes or until soft. Serve with the remaining juices, reduced, with a squeeze of lemon. You can also use fennel wedges, chicory (cut in half), leek or celery (cut into 10-cm lengths).

COURGETTE

Grate or finely slice (in rings) 1 courgette and mix with a squeeze of lemon juice, a splash of olive oil, a sprinkle of chilli flakes and chopped mint leaves or ¼ cup (25 g) of grated pecorino or parmesan.

PAK CHOI + SUGAR SNAP PEAS

Stir-fry ½ bunch of pak choi (each frond cut in half diagonally), ½ cup (50 g) of sugar snap peas with 1 finely chopped clove garlic and a splash of tamari, soy or Teriyaki Sauce (see page 206). Throw in 1 tablespoon of cashews.

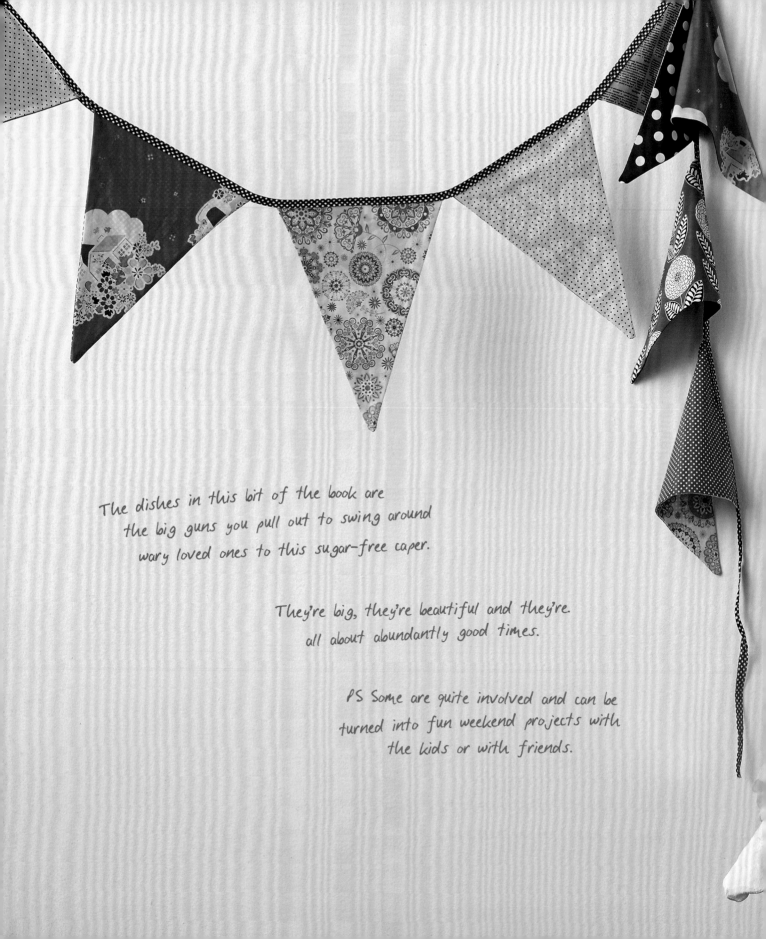

The dishes in this bit of the book are
the big guns you pull out to swing around
wary loved ones to this sugar-free caper.

They're big, they're beautiful and they're
all about abundantly good times.

PS Some are quite involved and can be
turned into fun weekend projects with
the kids or with friends.

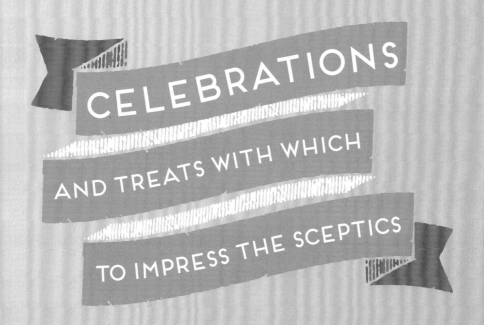

CELEBRATIONS

AND TREATS WITH WHICH

TO IMPRESS THE SCEPTICS

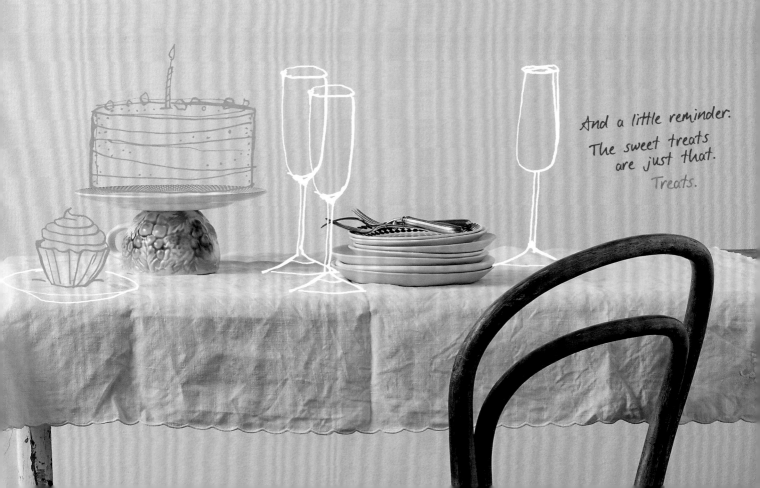

And a little reminder.
The sweet treats
are just that.
Treats.

LEMON MERINGUE PIES IN JARS

I know I seem a bit obsessed with Things In Jars, but bear with me: these pies really do work well in cute individual vessels, making them easy to tote to office morning teas and on picnics. You will need six 250-ml Mason jars for this recipe.

Preheat the oven to 160°C (gas 3) and line a baking tray with baking paper. To make the crumble base, start by throwing all the ingredients except for the water into a bowl or a food processor. Pulse with the food processor or rub with your fingers until the mixture resembles fine breadcrumbs. Add the water and continue to work the crumbs until small, chunky pieces of dough start to form. Spread them out on the prepared baking tray and bake for 15 minutes or until golden. Remove from the oven and allow to cool before processing again into rough crumbs. Leave the oven on.

While the crumble chunks are baking, make the lemon custard. Place the egg yolks, egg and stevia in a dry, heatproof bowl set over a saucepan of simmering water (the water should not touch the base of the bowl, and the bowl should fit snugly over the saucepan). Whisk until the stevia is dissolved and the eggs are lightly beaten, about 30 seconds. Add the lemon zest and juice and continue to whisk for 5–8 minutes, or until the custard is thick enough that when you draw a line with the whisk the line stays. Remove the bowl from the pan and set the custard aside to cool slightly. Once cool enough to touch, add the butter and whisk until melted through.

To make the meringue, in another dry bowl whisk together the egg whites and syrup until stiff peaks form – a good test is to turn the bowl upside down for a couple of seconds (carefully at first!) and if the meringue stays in the bowl, it's ready.

Place one-sixth of the crumble in the base of each jar. Top each base with about 4 tablespoons of the lemon custard and a good dollop of the meringue, to about the neck of the jar. Place the jars on a baking tray and bake for 10–12 minutes or until the meringue tops are starting to turn golden. Serve warm or cool, or screw on the lid and tote.

CRUMBLE BASE
¾ cup (85 g) plain flour or gluten-free plain flour

1 tablespoon granulated stevia

½ teaspoon ground ginger

1 teaspoon vanilla powder

50 g cold unsalted butter, diced

3 tablespoons water

LEMON CUSTARD
6 egg yolks (reserve 2 whites for Meringue)

1 egg

1½ tablespoons granulated stevia

grated zest and strained juice of 2 lemons

100 g unsalted butter

MERINGUE
2 egg whites (reserved from Custard)

2 tablespoons rice malt syrup

USING YOUR EGG WHITES
The remaining 4 raw egg whites can be stored in the fridge for a few days, covered with clingfilm, or frozen. They are perfect for eggy muggins, omelettes and scrambles.

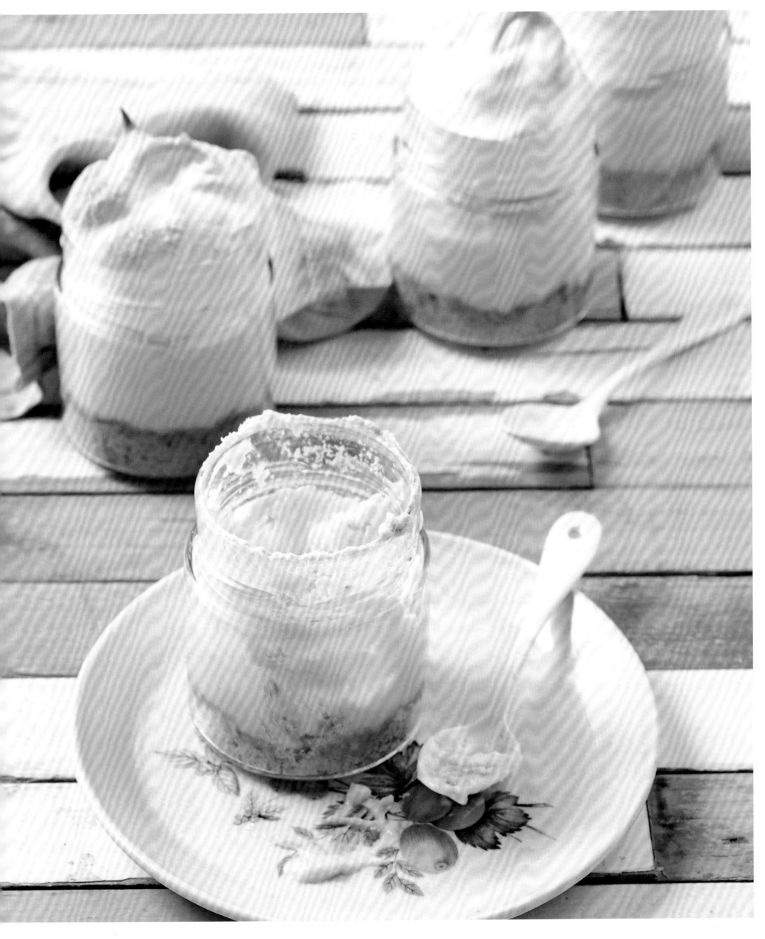

'NO-MORE-MUFFINS' *Meeting Treats*

Somewhat oddly, I'm often asked for ideas for fructose-free office morning teas. These suggestions are very multi-taskable. Cart them to picnics, afternoon teas at your best mate's place, Mum's house when you go to visit . . .

CHOC MINT SLICE

MAKES 25

To make the base, preheat the oven to 180°C (gas 4) and line a 20-cm square baking tin with baking paper. Combine the almond meal, cacao, arrowroot and baking powder in a bowl. Whisk together the eggs, syrup and water, then pour into the dry ingredients and mix well. Pour the batter into the prepared tin and bake for 20 minutes or until cooked. Set aside to cool completely on a wire rack.

To make the mint filling, pulse the shredded coconut with the boiling water and peppermint extract in a food processor until the mixture resembles breadcrumbs. Add the coconut oil and continue to pulse until combined. Press the mixture onto the cooled base and refrigerate for about 30 minutes, or freeze for about 10 minutes, to set.

To make the ganache topping, bring the cream to a simmer in a small saucepan. Remove from the heat and add the chopped chocolate, whisking well until all the chocolate is melted. Set aside to cool and thicken slightly. When the ganache has cooled, you may need to whisk it again briefly before pouring it over the mint filling. Return to the fridge until set. Cut into squares before serving.

BASE
2¼ cups (225 g) almond meal

⅓ cup (30 g) raw cacao powder

¼ cup (30 g) arrowroot

2 teaspoons baking powder

3 eggs

⅓ cup (75 ml) rice malt syrup

¼ cup (60 ml) water

MINT FILLING
3 cups (300 g) shredded coconut

2 tablespoons boiling water

1 tablespoon peppermint extract

½ cup (115 g) coconut oil, melted

GANACHE TOPPING
½ (125 ml) cup cream

100 g dark (85% cocoa) chocolate, roughly chopped

6 more *Wow-the-chick-from-Finance ideas*

LEMON MERINGUE PIES IN JARS (page 132)
Divide the mixture among smaller jars, or use small glasses.

FESTIVE POPCORN (page 148)
Serve in some fun cones or in a big bowl in the middle (where the lollies usually go!).

NUTTY CHEESE AND BACON LOLLIPOPS (page 159)
A very 'novelty' option, serve these stabbed into a big wheel of cheese (which you can eat after with some crackers).

FENNEL TARTE TATIN (page 127)
Sweet or savoury will work well; sprinkle with edible flowers for extra pizzazz!

NOT-QUITE-APPLE-CRUMBLE MUFFINS (page 62)
Serve warm.

OH-OH OREOS (page 184)
Or pretty much anything from the chocolate chapter.

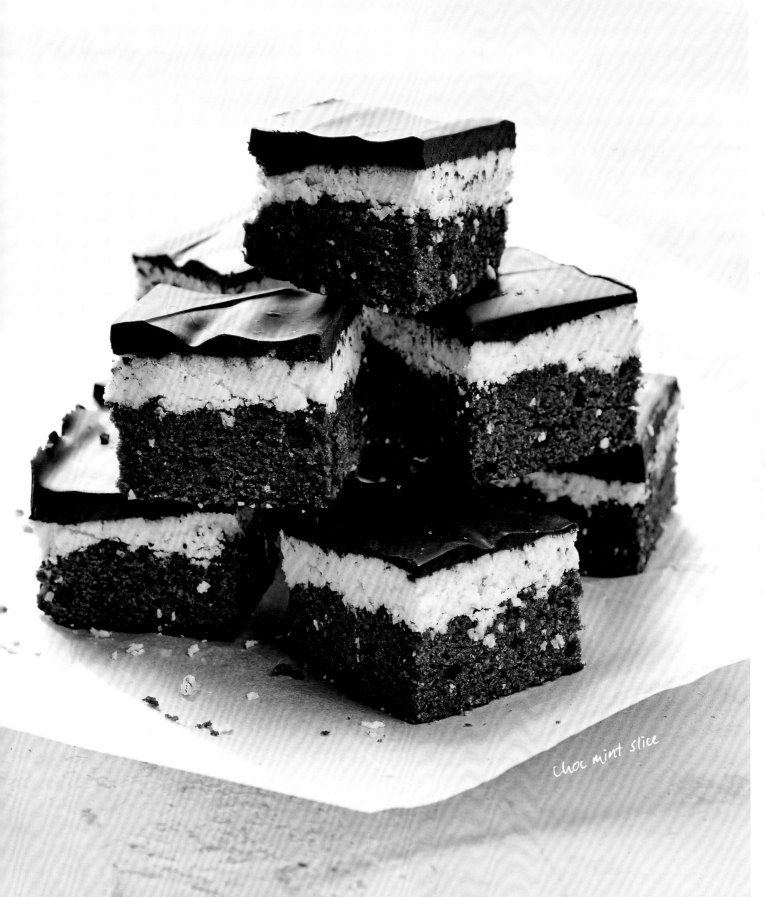

choc mint slice

ICE CREAM SUNDAE BIRTHDAY CAKE

A confession: this cake is a lot of trouble. It will take about 2 hours to make, not including the time it takes to make the Oreos, Strawberry Jam, Praline, Meringue, Ice Magic and Gooey Caramel Sauce. But it is a good one to build with the kids. Feel free to double the meringue quantity to make into additional party treats. It's best to make the cake on the day so that it stays cold and creamy.

First, make the Oreo base. Line the base of a 20-cm spring-form tin with baking paper. Pulse the Oreos in a food processor and transfer to the tin. Press evenly into the base and pop in the freezer for 10 minutes or until set.

Next, whip the cream with the stevia and vanilla powder until stiff peaks form. Keep the whipped cream in the fridge until you need it – you will be using a quarter of the mixture at a time.

To make the chocolate layer, combine all the ingredients except the Praline in a blender or using a stick blender until smooth. Add the Praline, then fold in one-quarter of the whipped cream thoroughly. Remove the tin from the freezer and pour the chocolate layer over the Oreo base, spreading it out evenly. Return it to the freezer for 15 minutes to set while you prepare the coconut vanilla layer.

To make the coconut vanilla layer, mix the coconut cream with the desiccated coconut, then fold through one-quarter of the whipped cream. Remove the tin from the freezer and pour the mixture over the chocolate layer, spreading it out evenly as before. Return the tin to the freezer for another 15 minutes.

To make the berry layer, remove the tin from the freezer and spread with the jam, then return to the freezer to set. Blend the berries, coconut cream and stevia in a blender or using a stick blender. Fold in one-quarter of the whipped cream and the meringue pieces, if using. Remove the tin from the freezer and pour the berry mixture over the coconut vanilla layer, spreading it out evenly. Return the cake to the freezer for about 1 hour or until set.

When you are ready to serve, remove the cake from the freezer and transfer it to a serving plate. Leave to stand for 10 minutes (about 5 minutes in hot weather). Transfer the remaining whipped cream to a piping bag or a sandwich bag with a corner snipped off, and pipe around the top. Arrange the raspberries on the cream. Drizzle over the Ice Magic. Drizzle the gooey caramel over the top.

BASE
1 quantity Oh-Oh Oreos (see page 184)

WHIPPED CREAM
3 cups (750 ml) cream

2 tablespoons granulated stevia

1 tablespoon vanilla powder

CHOCOLATE LAYER
1 small avocado

¾ cup (180 ml) coconut cream

1 tablespoon granulated stevia

2 tablespoons raw cacao powder

1 teaspoon vanilla powder

2 tablespoons Praline (see page 140)

COCONUT VANILLA LAYER
½ cup (125 ml) coconut cream

1½ tablespoons desiccated coconut

BERRY LAYER
½ cup (150 g) Strawberry Jam (see page 207)

2 cups (300 g) pre-cut and frozen strawberries or blueberries

¾ cup (180 ml) coconut cream

½ tablespoon granulated stevia

a handful of broken-up sugar-free meringue pieces (see page 144, optional)

TOPPING
12–14 raspberries

4 tablespoons Ice Magic (see page 180)

1 quantity Gooey Caramel Sauce (see page 140)

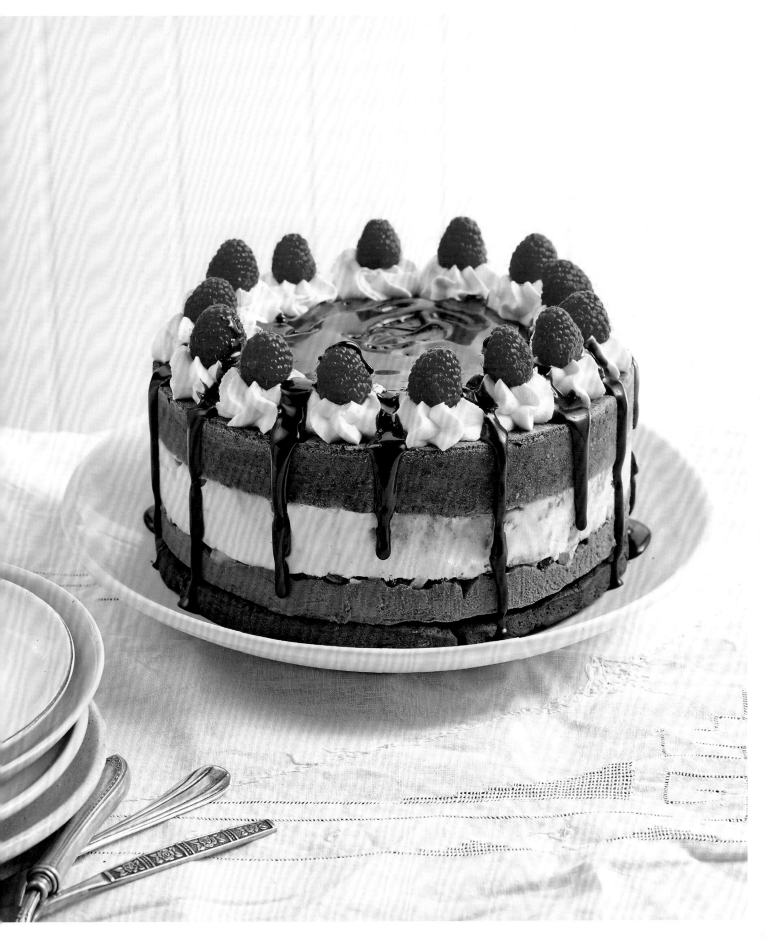

PIMP-MY-SPONGE EASTER CAKE

This cake takes a simple sponge recipe and jazzes it up in fun, fructose-free directions that can be rolled out for Easter or a kids' party. Of course, feel free to keep things simple and serve the basic sponge cake with whipped cream and my Strawberry Jam or fresh berries.

To make the nest, whisk together the egg whites and syrup, then fold in the coconut, quinoa and salt. Refrigerate for 1 hour.

To make the sponge, preheat the oven to 160°C (gas 3). Grease the sides of a 20-cm spring-form tin, dust with extra flour, then line the base with baking paper. Melt the butter and syrup in a small saucepan over low heat – do not boil – then set aside to cool slightly. Beat the eggs until light and fluffy. Sift the flour into a large bowl, then add the stevia and the melted butter and syrup mixture. Mix well. Add the eggs and fold to combine. Pour the batter into the prepared tin and bake in the centre of the oven for 30–35 minutes. Remove from the oven and cool in the tin for 10 minutes before transferring to a wire rack.

Wash each eggshell half thoroughly under warm running water, removing any membrane stuck to the inside. Pat dry, inside and out, with kitchen paper. Return the eggshell halves to the carton and pour in the chocolate. Refrigerate or freeze until set.

Remove the nest mixture from the fridge and line a baking tray with baking paper. Scoop the mixture onto the sheet and shape into a mound about 15 cm in diameter. Bake in the oven for 20 minutes or until golden brown. Set aside to cool, then refrigerate until ready to serve the cake.

Slice the cooled sponge in half horizontally and set aside the top half. Spread the jam over the bottom half, then replace the top half. Whip the cream with the stevia until stiff peaks form, then use to ice the sponge all over. Place the nest on top of the cake and pop some chocolate eggshells in the nest. Decorate with fluffy chicks, to serve.

NEST
3 egg whites

⅓ cup (75 ml) rice malt syrup

1½ cups (150 g) shredded coconut

1 cup (135 g) cooked quinoa (see page 94)

pinch of sea salt

SPONGE
200 g unsalted butter, plus extra for greasing

¼ cup (60 ml) rice malt syrup

4 eggs (retain the cracked eggshell halves for decoration)

200 g self-raising flour, plus extra for dusting

2 tablespoons granulated stevia

DECORATIONS
1 quantity Basic Raw Chocolate (see page 175)

1 cup (300 g) Strawberry Jam (see page 207)

1½ cups (350 ml) cream

1 teaspoon granulated stevia

mini fluffy toy chicks, to decorate

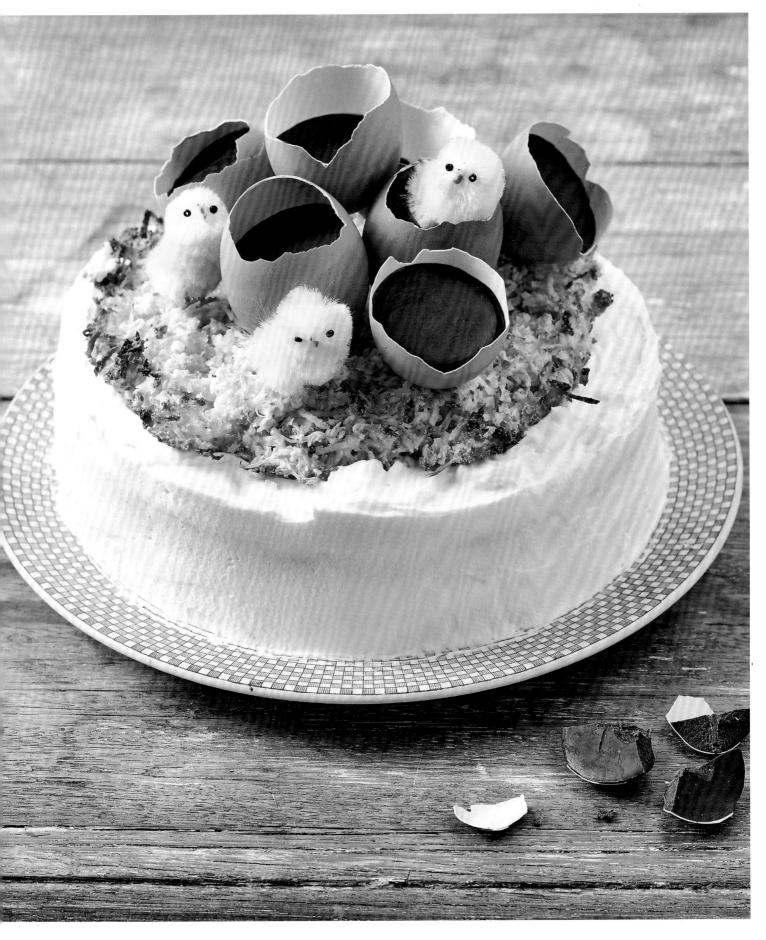

CHOC-CARAMEL-CHUNK AND PEANUT BUTTER 'CHEESECAKE'

 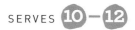

I wanted to create a party-stopping, ultra-indulgence, capable of inciting the most hardened sweet tooth to cry out, 'I can't believe THAT'S not sugar.' This was the result. Be warned: it is super-rich (albeit dense in nutrients) and sweet (albeit via the coco-nuttiness). So it should be treated as . . . a treat, OK? (Take note of the servings.)

Line the bottom and sides of a 23-cm spring-form tin with baking paper, then start by making the crust. Pulse the pecans in a food processor until roughly chopped. Add the remaining ingredients and process until the mixture has a moist, crumbly consistency. Spoon the mixture into the prepared tin and spread evenly around the base and 5 cm up the sides. Place in the fridge or freezer to set.

To make the caramel sauce, melt the butter with the syrup in a small saucepan over high heat. Bring to the boil, then reduce the heat to medium so that the mixture keeps bubbling – do not stir or the caramel will split. Cook for a further 4 minutes or until the caramel has turned golden and appears gooey when dripping off the back of a spoon. Remove from the heat and add the coconut cream, stirring gently. Transfer to a bowl and allow to cool.

To make the praline, preheat the grill to high and line a baking tray with baking paper. Warm the syrup gently, then mix with the nuts and transfer to the prepared tray. Grill for 5 minutes or until most of the water has evaporated and the syrup has turned golden and crystallised around the nuts. Remove from the grill and cool, then smash the praline into small pieces. Reserve 8 tablespoons for the topping, and keep the rest for the ice-cream filling.

To make the ice-cream filling, pulse the cashews with ⅓ cup (75 ml) of the coconut cream in a food processor until the mixture is smooth and buttery. Transfer to a large bowl and set aside. Again using the food processor, pulse the avocados with the remaining coconut cream, the cacao, salt and stevia until smooth. Add to the cashew mixture, then add the cinnamon, peanut butter, cacao nibs and praline. Stir well to combine.

[recipe continues over page]

CRUST
4½ cups (500 g) pecans

2 tablespoons raw cacao powder

1½ tablespoons coconut oil, melted

3 teaspoons vanilla powder or extract

1½ tablespoons rice malt syrup

GOOEY CARAMEL SAUCE
100 g butter, chopped

½ cup (125 ml) rice malt syrup

⅔ cup (150 ml) coconut cream

PRALINE
½ cup (125 ml) rice malt syrup

1 cup (225 g) peanuts or macadamia nuts, or both, roughly chopped

ICE-CREAM FILLING
3 cups (450 g) raw unsalted cashews

1¼ cups (300 ml) coconut cream

3 small avocados

⅓ cup (30 g) raw cacao powder

1½ teaspoons sea salt

1½ tablespoons granulated stevia

¾ teaspoon ground cinnamon

1½ cups (340 g) natural, sugar-free and salt-free crunchy peanut butter

1½ tablespoons cacao nibs

CHOCOLATE SAUCE
¼ cup (50 g) coconut oil

1½ tablespoons rice malt syrup

1½ tablespoons raw cacao powder

small pinch of sea salt

1 tablespoon coconut cream

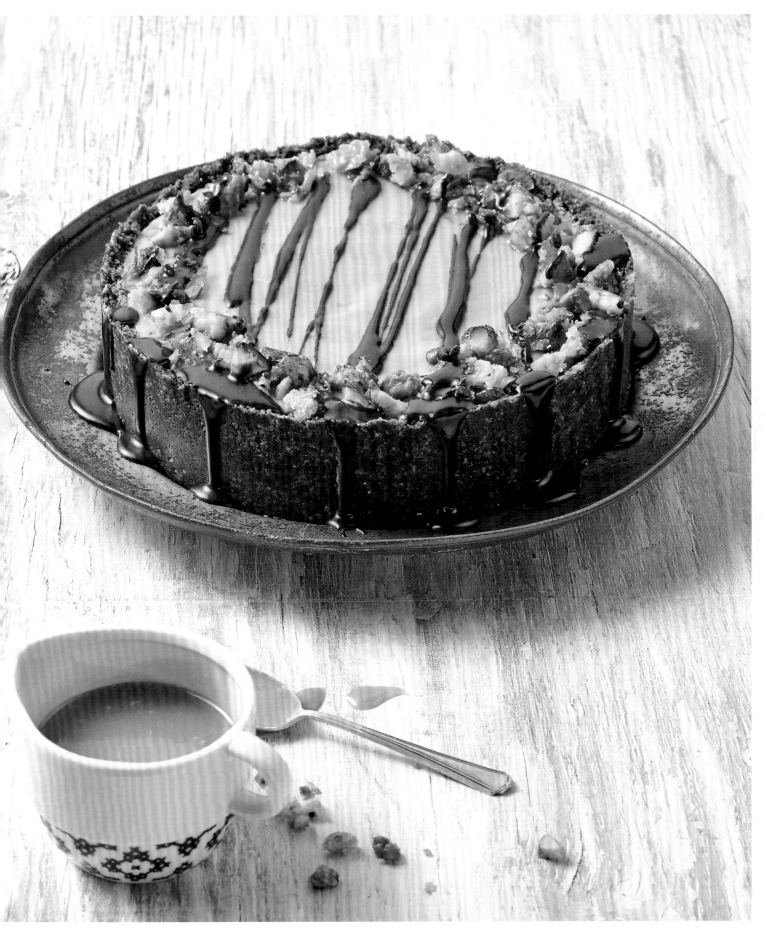

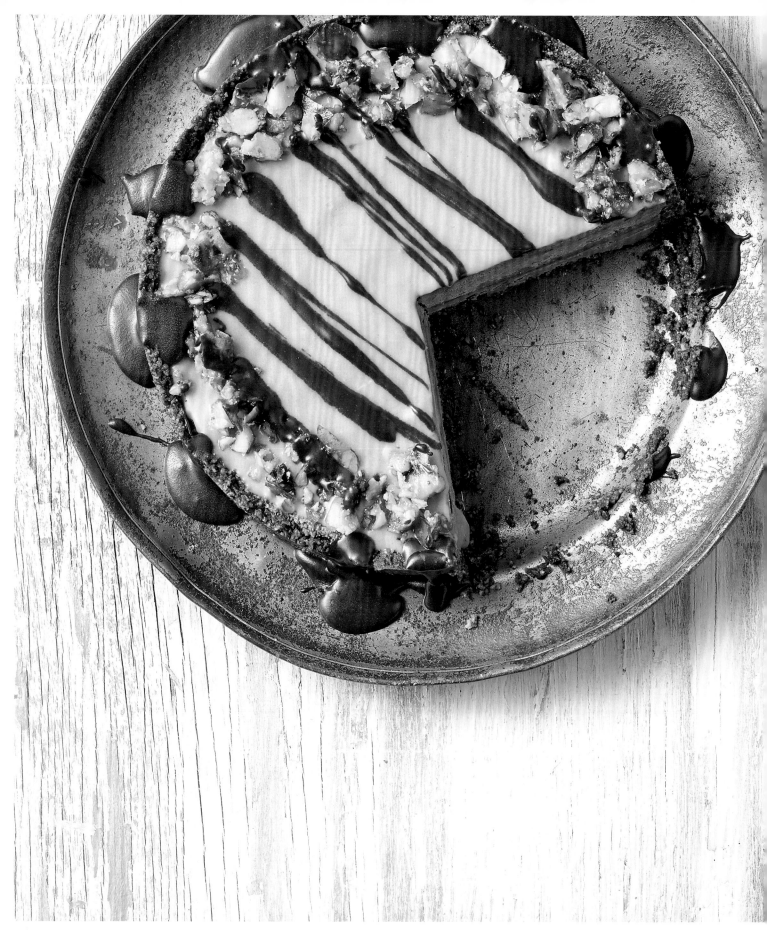

Spoon about half of the ice-cream mixture over the crust in the spring-form tin and spread right to the edges of the crust. Freeze for 5–10 minutes, then drizzle over half the caramel sauce. Freeze for another 5–10 minutes, then add the remaining ice-cream mixture. Freeze for 5–10 minutes, then add the remaining caramel sauce and freeze the assembled cake for at least 6 hours, or overnight.

To make the chocolate sauce, throw the coconut oil and syrup into a small saucepan and melt together over low heat. Remove from the heat and whisk through the cacao powder and salt until thoroughly combined, with no lumps. Leave to cool for 5 minutes, then whisk through the coconut cream until smooth. (This sauce will thicken as it cools and can be reheated to make it runnier.) If the mixture makes more sauce then you need, just pour it into moulds and make some chocolates.

To serve, remove the cake from the freezer and the tin and transfer to a serving plate. Arrange the reserved praline around the edge of the plate and drizzle over the chocolate sauce. Allow to stand for 5 minutes before serving.

VEGAN: Amend the Gooey Caramel Sauce. Place ¼ cup (60 ml) rice malt syrup and ½ cup (125 ml) coconut cream in a saucepan and bring to the boil over high heat. Reduce the heat to medium and continue to boil for about 6 minutes or until the sauce has thickened and is gooey. It will keep for 5 days in the fridge.

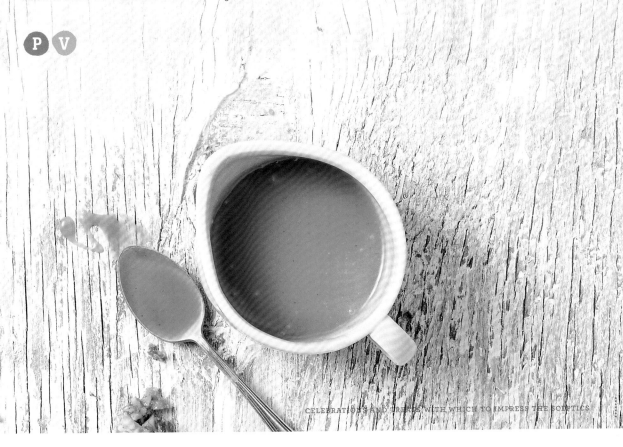

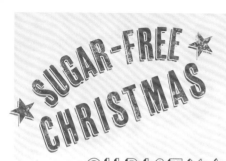

CHRISTMAS PAVLOVA TRIFLE

SERVES **8**

I've included a few sugar-free Christmas ideas here and have designed them so that much of the dish can be prepared in advance to save you sweating it out in the kitchen on Christmas Day. Pork neck is a fantastic alternative to sugar and nitrate-laden store-bought hams, with a texture somewhere between ham and roasted meat.

Christmas Eve: Start by making the meringues. Preheat the oven to 120°C (gas ½) and line a baking tray with baking paper. Beat the egg whites with the salt to form stiff peaks. Add the syrup, if using, and beat a little more. Stop beating and gently fold in the coconut. Form mixture into rough balls, then arrange on the prepared tray and bake for 30 minutes. Reduce oven temperature to 95°C (lowest gas setting) and bake for another hour, by which time the meringues will be chewy. Bake for several hours more if you like them crispy. Remove from the oven and set aside to cool completely before removing them from the baking paper. Store in an airtight container overnight.

Meanwhile, make a simple coulis by mixing the berries with the stevia, then bringing to a gentle boil and reducing for a few minutes. Store in the fridge overnight.

Christmas Day: Roughly crumble 12 meringues and set aside. Whip the coconut cream or milk with the yoghurt or cream cheese and the salt until thick. Arrange the crumbled meringue chunks (reserving a few for topping) in the bottom of 8 glasses (mugs or cocktail stems could also work). Divide three-quarters of the berries among 8 glasses, then place a big dollop of cream on top of each. Arrange the remaining berries and meringue chunks on top and serve.

(P)

MERINGUES
4 egg whites

pinch of sea salt

⅓ cup (75 ml) rice malt syrup (optional)

2½ cups (250 g) shredded coconut

COULIS
1½ cups (225 g) frozen berries

2 teaspoons granulated stevia

400 ml can coconut cream or milk, chilled in the fridge

1½ cups (350 ml) full-fat organic plain yoghurt or 350 g Homemade Cream Cheese (see page 204)

pinch of sea salt

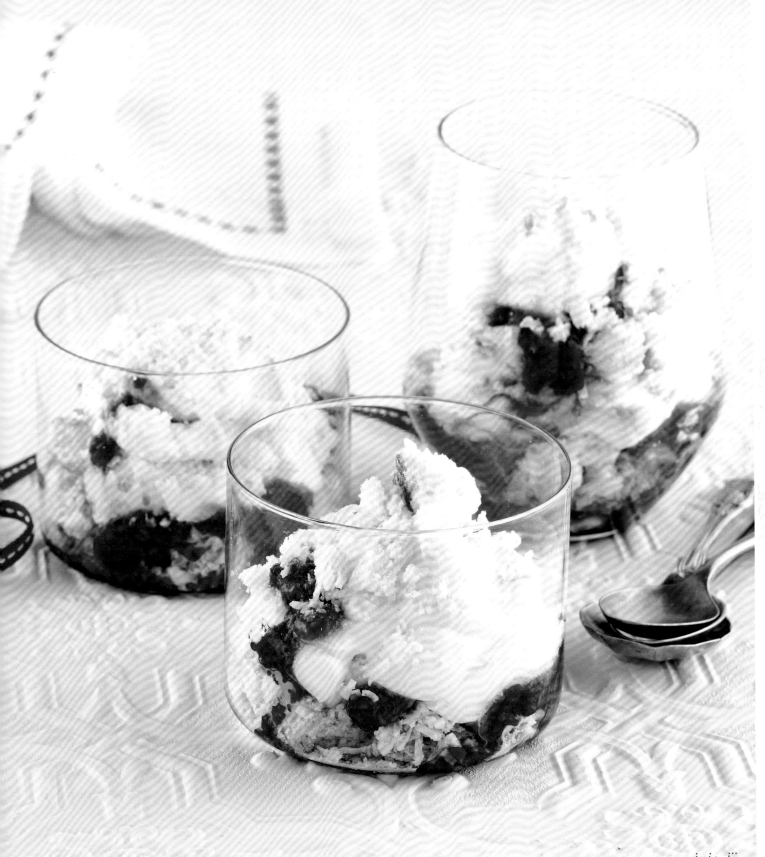

★ CHRISTMAS 'MAPLE HAM'

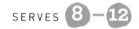

SERVES 8 – 12

Christmas Eve: Line a large baking dish with baking paper. Wash the pork under cold running water and pat dry with kitchen paper. Place the pork, fat-marbled side up, in the prepared baking dish. Mix the spices, salt, pepper, syrup, olive oil, water, and orange zest and juice in a jug and pour over the pork, rubbing well into the meat. Cover and marinate in the fridge for at least 8 hours or overnight.

Christmas Day: Preheat the oven to 200°C (gas 6). Remove the pork from the fridge and allow to stand for 10 minutes. Add ½ cup (125 ml) water to the base of the dish and pop the lot in the oven. Bake for 30 minutes then turn the baking dish around and bake for a further 30 minutes, adding another ½ cup (125 ml) of water if necessary. Bake for a further 30 minutes, turning the dish around after 15 minutes. Serve warm on its own or with relish, Stuffins, and your choice of vegetables.

2 kg piece of boneless pork neck

1 tablespoon paprika

2 teaspoons ground cloves

1 teaspoon ground cinnamon

1 teaspoon sea salt

1 teaspoon freshly ground black pepper

½ cup (125 ml) rice malt syrup

4 tablespoons olive oil

4 tablespoons water

grated zest of 1 orange

2 tablespoons orange juice

Beetroot and Apple relish (see page 199), Stuffins (see page 147) and steamed greens (see pages 128–9), to serve

---

★ YULE MULE COCKTAILS

MAKES APPROXIMATELY 10 DRINKS

The perfect gut-grounding tipple for the silly season. Please note: you'll need to prepare the base Gingerade recipe a week in advance of Christmas Day.

Christmas Day: Juice 4 of the limes and add to the vodka in a jug. Combine the Gingerade and soda in another jug. Cut remaining 2 limes into small wedge-like chunks. Half-fill tall glasses with crushed ice and lime wedges. Then pour ⅓ cup (75 ml) of the vodka and lime over the top, then top with Gingerade mixture. Serve.

6 limes

500 ml vodka

crushed ice

1 litre Gingerade (see page 203)

1 litre soda water

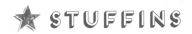
These stuffing muffins are a novel way to do stuffing and don't contain any dried fruit.

Christmas Eve: Grease two 8-cup muffin tins with the oil, butter or ghee and line the tins. Heat a frying pan over medium–high heat and sauté the pancetta or sausage until slightly browned. Transfer to kitchen paper to drain. Using the same pan (and the pancetta fat), sauté the celery and onion with the butter until they caramelise. Remove from the heat and stir in the pancetta or sausage, bread, lemon zest and parsley. Lightly beat the eggs with the milk, then pour over the top. Add the chicken stock a little at a time and mix gently. Keep adding stock until everything is definitely moist (but not soggy). Season with salt and pepper, spoon the mixture into the prepared muffin tins and refrigerate overnight.

Christmas Day: Preheat the oven to 200°C (gas 6) or pop into the oven if you are already cooking the ham in the final part of the ham's cooking process. Bake the muffins for 30–40 minutes or until cooked and lightly browned.

coconut oil, butter or ghee, for greasing

500 g pancetta, diced, or
    500 g gourmet pork sausages, sliced

2 celery stalks, chopped

1 onion, chopped

1 tablespoon butter

1 loaf bread (any kind), thickly sliced,
    cut into 2-cm dice and toasted in a
    150°C (gas 2) oven for 10 minutes

grated zest of 1 lemon

1 cup (30 g) chopped flat-leaf parsley

3 eggs

½ cup (125 ml) milk

3 cups (750 ml) Leftovers Chicken Stock
    (see page 191)

sea salt and freshly ground black pepper

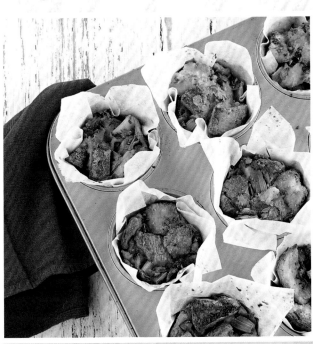

FESTIVE POPCORN

MAKES ABOUT 8 CUPS (90 G)

In a very big saucepan with a lid, heat the oil over high heat and cook the popcorn (with the lid on), shaking the pan often. Once you hear the last of the kernels pop, remove from the heat. Place the popcorn in a large saucepan. Melt the butter with the spices, salt and syrup in a small saucepan and pour over the popcorn. Stir thoroughly. Serve warm or cold.

NOTE: If you're making these for a party, prepare the popcorn the night before, cool and store in an airtight container. The next day you complete the butter and spices stage.

2 tablespoons coconut or olive oil

¾ cup (160 g) popcorn kernels

½ cup (115 g) butter

5 teaspoons ras el hanout
   (or 2 teaspoons each of ground cinnamon,
   cumin and cayenne pepper)

1 tablespoon sea salt

2 tablespoons rice malt syrup

ANZAC BISCUITS

MAKES 16

For anyone outside Australia and New Zealand, let me tell you about Anzac biscuits. They were eaten by our soldiers in World War I in lieu of bread and were a rock-hard combo of long-lasting foods that could withstand the journey via ship to reach the troops: oats, flour, golden syrup, coconut and bicarbonate of soda. They had a crook reputation for cracking a few teeth, so some of the wives and mums back home decided to finesse things a little. Today we make them to remember the fallen – and because they taste great.

Preheat the oven to 180°C (gas 4) and line a baking tray with baking paper. Mix the flour, stevia, coconut, vanilla, cinnamon and oats in a bowl. In a small saucepan, melt the butter and syrup together until the mixture starts to bubble, then stir through the bicarbonate of soda. Add the lot to the bowl and stir to combine. Roll heaped teaspoonfuls of the mixture into balls and flatten on the baking tray. Bake for 15 minutes or until golden brown. Cool completely on the baking tray on a rack to ensure they turn crispy!

PALEO: Replace the flour with quinoa and the oats with ½ cup (50 g) of almond meal.

¾ cup (85 g) plain flour

⅓ cup (75 g) granulated stevia

¾ cup (75 g) desiccated coconut

½ teaspoon vanilla powder

½ teaspoon ground cinnamon

¾ cup (75 g) rolled oats

100 g salted butter

2 tablespoons rice malt syrup

½ teaspoon bicarbonate of soda,
   dissolved in 1 tablespoon boiling water

I QUIT SUGAR FOR LIFE

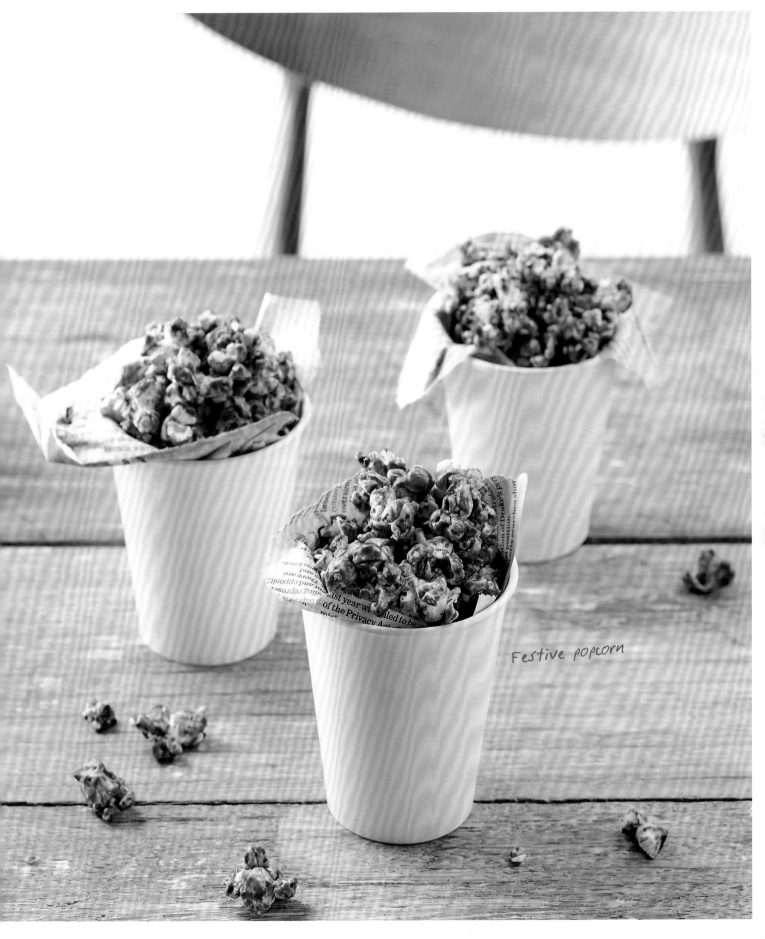

Festive popcorn

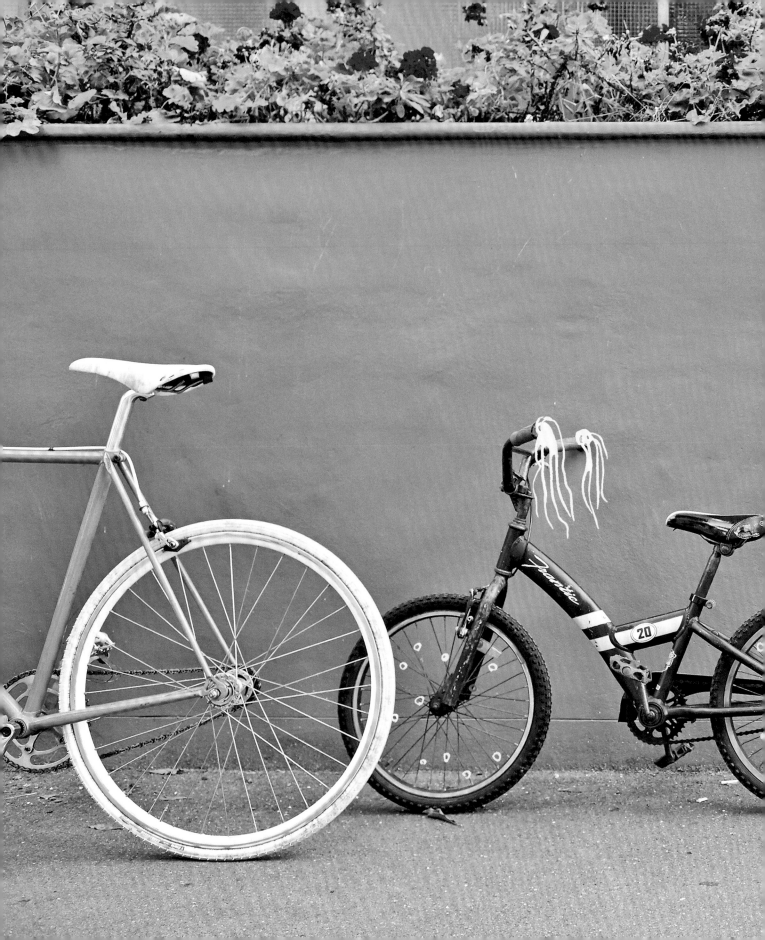

KIDS' LUNCHES AND SNACKS

How to get kids on board the sugar-free, nutrient-dense train? Hmmm, a few things...

1. Try not to stigmatise sugar (rather than 'ban' it, just don't have it in the house).

2. Take your kids to do the grocery shopping and have them help you find the best sugar-free, nutrient-dense options.

3. Get them involved in the cooking. Or the growing. Just get them fired up about good food!

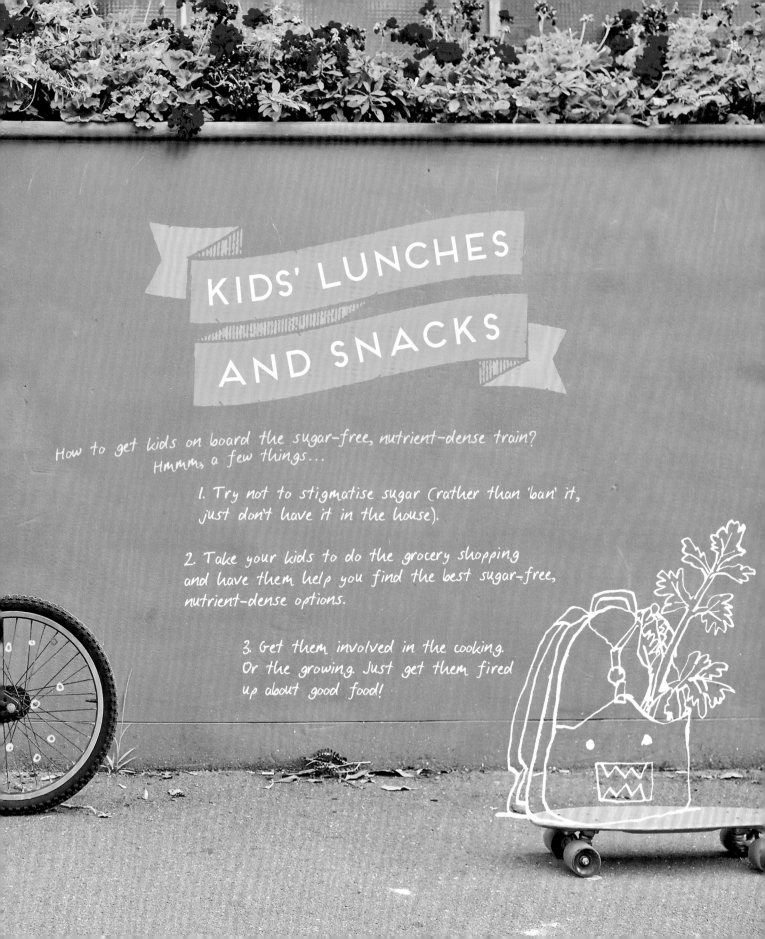

LCM BARS (AKA RICE KRISPIES SQUARES FOR YOU BRITS) MAKES

I've remodelled these very sugary snacks into less crappy versions, getting the caramel-y, marshmallow effect from the nuts and the rice malt syrup.

Line a 20-cm square baking tin with baking paper. Process the macadamias in a blender or using the chopper attachment of a stick blender for 3 minutes, or until the nuts form a smooth paste. Measure out ½ cup (125 g) of the macadamia paste and put in a large saucepan. (Any leftover macadamia butter will keep in an airtight container or jar in the fridge for up to 2 months.)

Toss the puffed rice cereal or popped corn into a large bowl. Add the syrup, vanilla and salt (if using) to the saucepan of macadamia butter and place over low heat. Cook, stirring constantly, until the mixture begins to 'melt'. Remove the pan from the heat and pour over the rice cereal or popped corn. Mix well, until each piece of puffed rice or popped corn is covered with the mixture. Press into the prepared tin, using the back of a spoon to push the mixture into the corners. Refrigerate for 15 minutes or until set. Slice into squares or bars and store in an airtight container in the fridge.

NOTE: If you use puffed brown rice, the bars will be chewy rather than crispy.

- 1 cup (225 g) macadamia nuts
- 4 cups (50 g) low-sugar puffed rice cereal or sugar-free puffed brown rice or popped corn
- ½ cup (125 ml) rice malt syrup
- 1 teaspoon vanilla powder
- 1½ teaspoons sea salt (optional, for salted caramel flavour)

I QUIT SUGAR FOR LIFE

Blythswood Trading Ltd
Thank You
Thank you!

CUSTOMER COPY

CARDNET

MID ****04593
TID ****5104   Receipt: 3567

2022-Jan-22   12:26:09

Sale

                                          VISA
VISA DEBIT   CONTACTLESS

446292******0138
PSN   00

AID   A0000000031010
ARQC   1943B5ED8D4C709F

TOTAL   £1.50

NO CARDHOLDER VERIFICATION
APPROVED

Visa Contactless

AUTH CODE <024334>

Please debit my account
with the total amount

PLEASE RETAIN RECEIPT

Thank you!

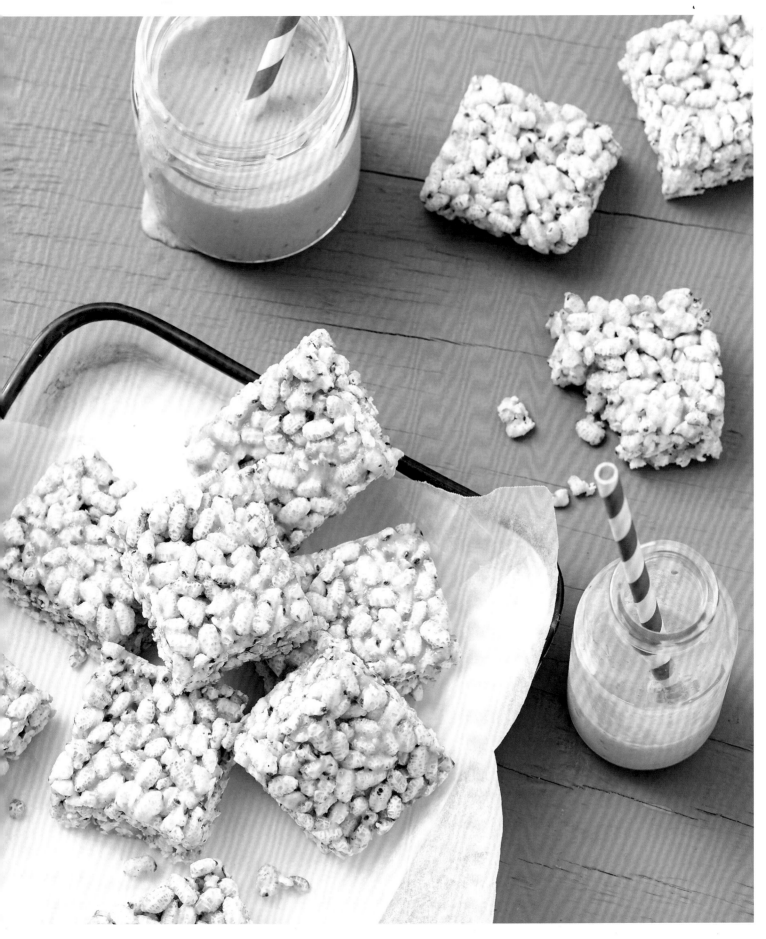

PUMPKIN CHEESECAKE LOLLIES

Blend all the ingredients in a blender or using a stick blender and pour into ice-lolly moulds. Insert the sticks and freeze for at least 4 hours.

1 cup (250 ml) full-fat organic plain yoghurt (Greek-style is best) or coconut yoghurt

1 cup (250 ml) coconut milk

1 teaspoon granulated stevia

1 cup (250 ml) Pumpkin Purée (see page 51)

2 teaspoons ground cinnamon

1 teaspoon ground allspice or nutmeg (optional)

MANGO WEIS-ISH BARS

MAKES 4—6

Re-own these nostalgic summer favourites. Eat sitting on a flaked-paint picnic bench outside the takeaway at your closest beachside caravan park if you like!

Blend the coconut cream, syrup and coconut in a blender or using a stick blender and pour into ice-lolly moulds until they're one-third full. Add a sprinkle of chopped macadamia nuts. Freeze for 1 hour. Add the mango to the remaining coconut mixture and blend. Top up the moulds with the mango mixture, insert the sticks and freeze for at least 4 hours.

400 ml can coconut cream

1 tablespoon rice malt syrup

⅓ cup (35 g) desiccated coconut

1 cup (120 g) frozen mango (pre-diced and frozen)

sprinkle of chopped macadamia nuts

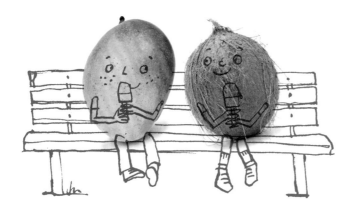

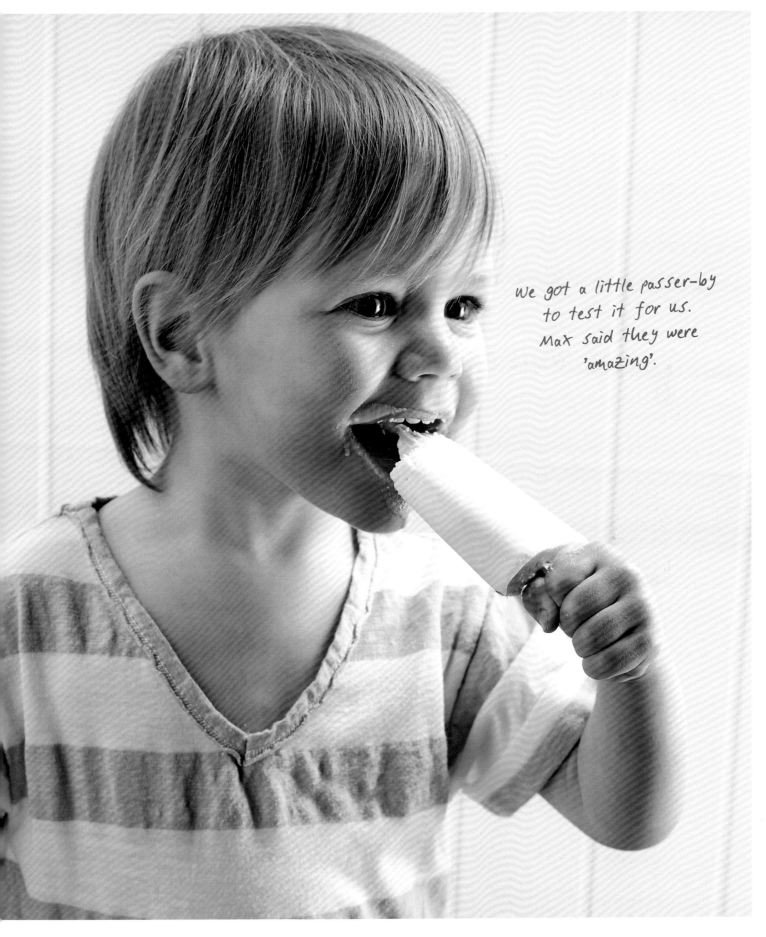

We got a little passer-by
to test it for us.
Max said they were
'amazing'.

Preheat the oven to 160°C (gas 3) and line a 20-cm square baking tin with baking paper. In a large bowl, mix together the nuts, oats and coconut flakes. In a saucepan, melt the oil or butter, syrup, Pumpkin Purée and spices. Add the chia seeds and bring the mixture to a gentle boil. Remove from the heat and stir through the nut and oat mixture until well combined, then continue mixing for another minute to help the ingredients bind. Press the mixture evenly into the prepared tin and bake for 30–40 minutes or until golden. Remove from the oven and allow to cool before slicing into bars. Store in an airtight container in a cool, dry place for 1–2 weeks.

PALEO: Replace oats with puffed quinoa or puffed rice.

Adult Variation:
PUMPKIN PROTEIN BARS
You can pump up the protein power further by adding ½ cup (50 g) vanilla protein powder to the dry mix.

- 2 cups (300 g) mixed almonds, cashews, pecans, walnuts and pumpkin seeds (preferably activated, see page 204), roughly chopped
- 2 cups (200 g) rolled oats
- 2 cups (150 g) coconut flakes
- 6 tablespoons coconut oil (or butter, or a mixture of both)
- ¾ cup (180 ml) rice malt syrup
- 1 cup (250 ml) Pumpkin Purée (see page 51)
- 1 teaspoon ground cinnamon
- 1 teaspoon ground allspice
- 1 teaspoon ground ginger
- ½ teaspoon ground cloves (optional)
- 5 tablespoons chia seeds

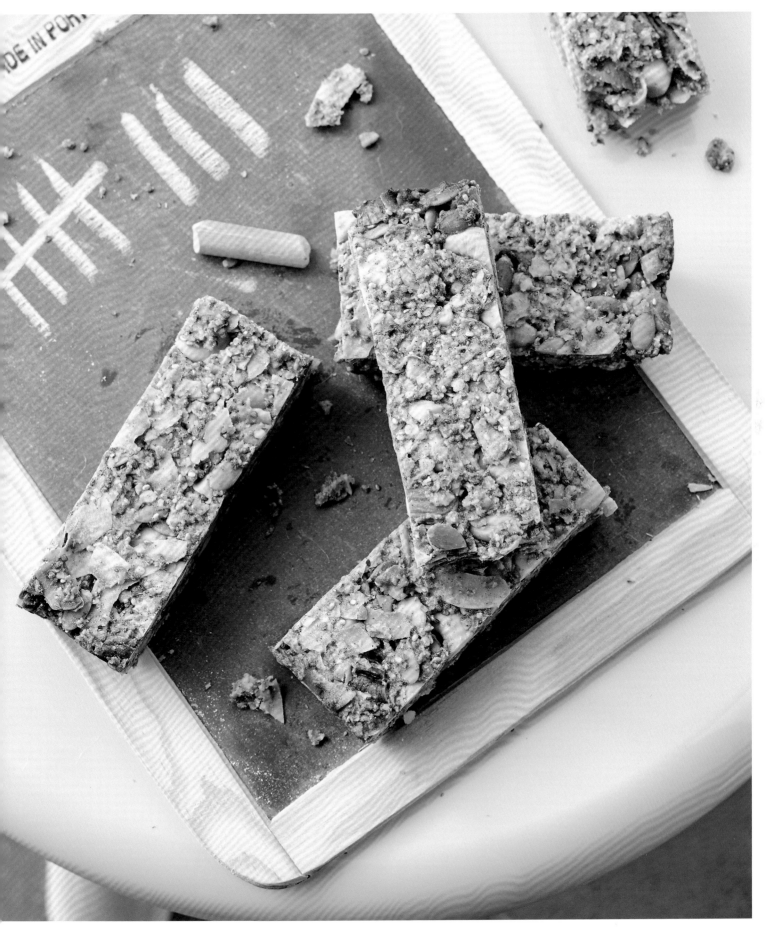

STUPIDLY SIMPLE SUGAR-FREE *Snack Ideas*

I really encourage keeping snacking as an occasional thing, for DVD days on the couch, hikes, road trips and the like. For such occasions you might like to try these five-ingredients-or-less ideas.

BOMBAY GRANOLA

MAKES ABOUT **5** CUPS (425 G)

Both this and the cheesy granola are great sprinkled on top of soups, or salads too.

Preheat the oven to 120°C (gas ½) and line a baking tray with baking paper. Combine all the ingredients except the egg white and tamari in a large bowl. In a small bowl, whisk together the egg white and tamari, then pour over the nut mixture and stir until combined. Spread the mixture out evenly on the prepared tray. Bake for 25 minutes, stirring at the 10-minute mark. Remove from the oven and allow to cool completely.

Lush Variation:
CHEESY GRANOLA

Omit the coconut flakes and curry powder and add 1 tablespoon of chopped thyme, 2 cups (200 g) of rolled oats, and ⅓ cup (40 g) of finely grated cheese (gruyere is the go).

- 3 cups (225 g) coconut flakes
- 2 cups (300 g) mixed almonds, cashews, pecans, walnuts and pumpkin seeds (preferably activated; see page 204), roughly chopped
- 2 tablespoons chia seeds
- 1 tablespoon curry powder
- ½ teaspoon cayenne pepper
- 1 teaspoon sea salt
- 1 teaspoon onion or garlic powder
- 80–100 g coconut oil or butter, melted
- 1 large egg white
- 1 teaspoon tamari

AVOCADO MOUSSE CAKES

MAKES **4**

Mash the avocado using the back of a fork. Add the lime zest and juice, syrup, vanilla and salt. Spread on rice cakes (toast lightly if you like) and sprinkle on coconut.

- 1 large avocado
- grated zest and juice of ½ lime
- 1 tablespoon rice malt syrup
- ½ teaspoon vanilla essence or a sprinkle of vanilla powder
- big pinch of salt
- 4 rice cakes, to serve
- coconut flakes or shredded coconut, to serve

NUTTY CHEESE AND BACON LOLLIPOPS

MAKES 8

Combine the cheeses, half the herbs, salt and pepper in a bowl. Divide into 8 bite-sized pieces, roll into balls and insert a bamboo skewer into each. Refrigerate overnight or freeze for 20 minutes. Meanwhile, cook the bacon until crispy. Allow to cool, then crumble up and mix with crushed nuts and the remaining herbs. Roll the balls in the bacon and nut mixture and serve.

Daggy Variation:

For a 1980s version: shape into a log and roll in the bacon and nut mixture. Wrap in greaseproof paper, refrigerate overnight, then serve with crackers!

P **8WP**

- ½ cup (115 g) Homemade Cream Cheese (see page 204)
- ½ cup (50 g) grated cheddar or crumbled goat's cheese
- 4 tablespoons chopped herbs (thyme or basil are great)
- sea salt and freshly ground black pepper
- 4 rashers bacon
- 3–4 tablespoons crushed pecans or almonds

THYME 'HONEY' HALOUMI

MAKES 1

This Greek dish is often served as a starter. I eat it as dessert.

Grill the haloumi on one side in a small frying pan over medium heat. When that side is browned, add the syrup, butter and herbs on top of the cheese, then flip the cheese and brown on the other side. Add the walnuts and cook until browned. Squeeze the lemon over the top and toss the pan until the sauce caramelises. Serve immediately.

P

- 2 slices haloumi
- ½ tablespoon rice malt syrup
- 1 teaspoon butter
- 1 teaspoon finely chopped thyme, rosemary or mint
- 1 tablespoon chopped walnuts
- small wedge of lemon

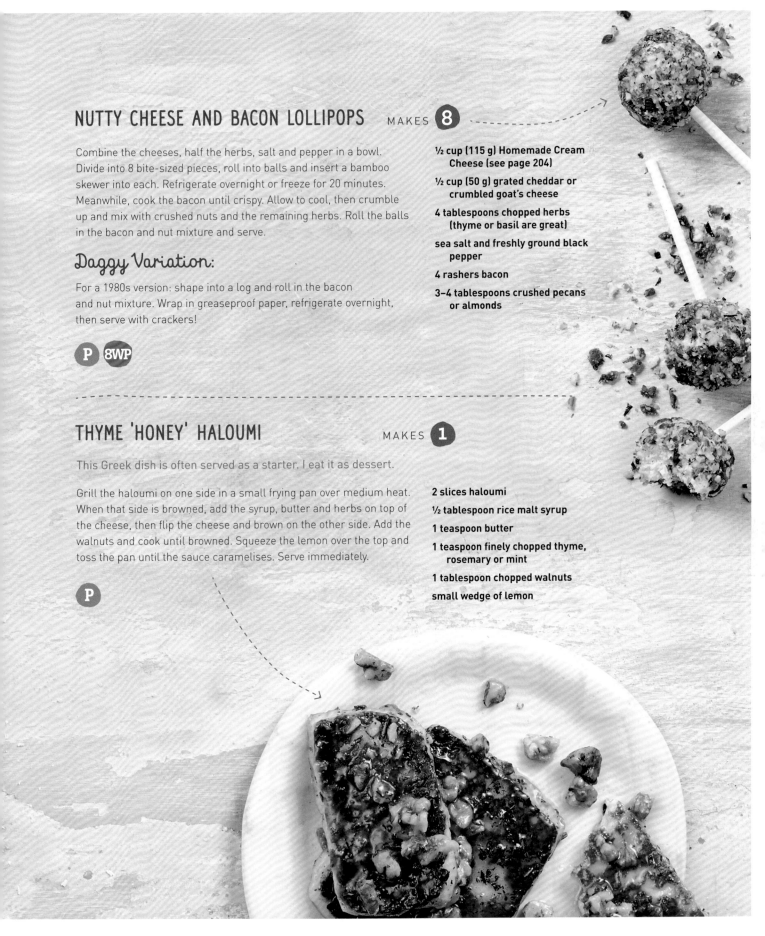

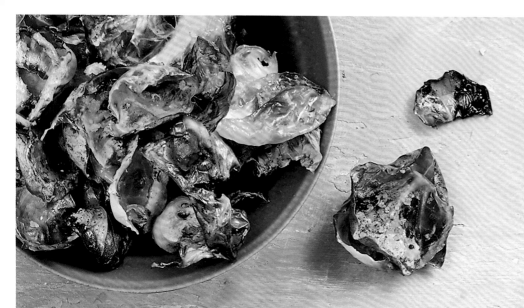

CRISPY BRUSSELS SPROUTS CHIPS

SERVES

Preheat the oven to 200ºC (gas 6) and line a baking tray with baking paper. Cut off the bottom tip of each sprout and peel off the leaves layer by layer. Toss the leaves with the oil until well coated and spread out in one layer on the prepared baking tray. Sprinkle with salt and bake for 8–10 minutes or until the leaves are lightly browned and crisp. Eat right away (they go soggy after a few hours).

NOTE: This is a great way to use up the outer leaves of your sprouts. I prefer to keep the 'hearts' and use only the outer leaves for these chips.

10 Brussels sprouts
1 tablespoon olive oil
¼ teaspoon sea salt

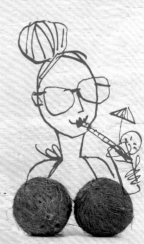

COCONUT CHAI FROZEN YOGHURT

SERVES

Blend the yoghurt, coconut milk and coconut in a blender or using a stick blender. Squeeze the chai tea bags and pour the steeped tea liquid over the mixture and stir. Freeze for 3 hours, then blend again briefly.

2 cups (500 ml) full-fat organic plain yoghurt
400 ml can coconut milk
1 cup (100 g) desiccated coconut
4 chai tea bags steeped in 2 tablespoons boiling water

PIMPED PEANUT BUTTER PUTTY

MAKES 1½ CUPS (350 ML)

Throw all the ingredients into a blender and blend until smooth. Pour into a jar and refrigerate until thick.

½ (115 g) cup natural, sugar-free and salt-free peanut butter

½ cup (125 ml) almond milk (or coconut or regular milk will do)

4 tablespoons vanilla protein powder

½ teaspoon ground cinnamon

1 tablespoon rice malt syrup

sea salt

Serving Ideas:

⁜ Spread on crackers with sliced Fermented Cucumbers (see page 199).

⁜ Put a splodge on top of your Up 'n' Go Breakfast Whip (see page 84) or Peanut Butter 'n' Jelly Porridge Whip (see page 75)

⁜ Drizzle over full-fat organic plain yoghurt or Whipped Coconut Cream (see page 72) or Pumpkin Pikelets (see page 191) with a splodge of Strawberry Jam (see page 207).

⁜ Eat as a dip with some apple slices.

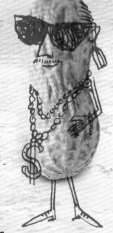

SALTED DARK CHOCOLATE POPCORN

SERVES 4

Cook the popcorn in a saucepan (see page 148), or in a lunch bag in the microwave (see page 168) with half the coconut oil. Mix the remaining coconut oil with the cacao, syrup and sea salt and then heat gently in a small saucepan or in the microwave until melted. Add to the cooked popcorn and toss to combine. Add salt, spread out on a small tray and refrigerate until firm.

NOTE: If you have some leftover Ice Magic (see page 180), you can use this instead of making the chocolate mixture from scratch. Feel free to add nut butter and cayenne pepper for extra fun. You can also bake the whole lot at 120°C (gas ½) for 30 minutes, stirring frequently, for a crispier version.

2 tablespoons popcorn kernels

2 tablespoons coconut oil

1½ tablespoons raw cacao powder

1 tablespoon rice malt syrup

large pinch of sea salt

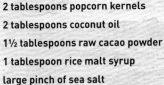

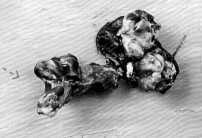

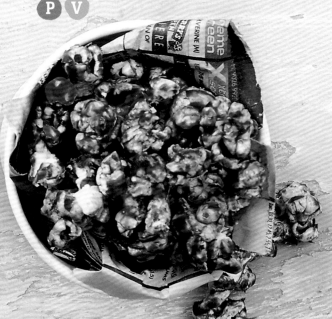

WEEKEND PRoJECT

Homemade Sprouts

A ripper way to get kids engaged in their food is to have them grow it. Sprouting is super simple and a perfect weekend project for little impatient beings – they'll be able to dine on their bounty by mid-week. The Chia Heads (over) are quite a lot of fun. I made them with my best mate's kids and was seriously surprised by their enthusiasm for the silliness.

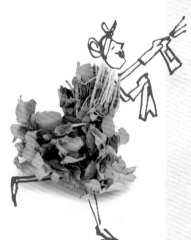

WHY THE SPROUTING?

Legumes, grains and seeds contain a host of toxins. It's natural, really. Animals have horns and teeth to defend themselves against predators. Legumes, grains and seeds have acids and dangerous enzyme inhibitors that keep us at bay by making us sick. Cultures around the world have overcome such a dietary annoyance by developing ways to change the chemical composition of these little life staples by sprouting them. Sprouting activates the seed's or grain's enzymes, which neutralise the harmful toxins, turning them into digestible and very much 'alive' food. It also creates extra vitamins and enzymes in the process. Furthermore, seeds are effectively plants – and plants are always alkalising.

And as I've mentioned before, sprouting slows ageing, which won't interest the kids so much . . . but you might like to know that activating the enzymes reduces the load on your body. Depletion of enzymes in the body is, in fact, the ageing process.

SPROUTED LEGUMES AND SEEDS

1 cup (200 g) dried legumes (chickpeas, brown lentils and mung beans work really well) or seeds (hulled sunflower seeds, pumpkin seeds)

You can buy a sprouting kit from garden centres and some health food shops. Or follow this method: first, get the kids to soak the legumes or seeds – simply dump the beans in a big bowl with plenty of water to cover. Have them pick out any 'floaters'. In the morning, drain and rinse in a wire sieve. Place the sieve over a bowl and put a saucepan lid on top. Leave on the worktop for 2–3 days (sunflower seeds only take 12–24 hours), and put the kids in charge of rinsing twice a day: rinse really well, filling the bowl with water up and over the legumes and stirring a little before draining. In summer, you'll need to rinse more often. White shoots will start to form after a day or so. Once they're about 5 mm long, store in an airtight container in the fridge.

BEWARE

DON'T GO OVERBOARD. YOU DON'T WANT TO EAT TOO MANY RAW SPROUTED LEGUMES. THEY STILL CONTAIN A FEW TOXINS . . . AND CAN BRING ON, UM, EXCESSIVE WIND IF CONSUMED IN BULK. THE BEST IDEA IS TO ALSO COOK YOUR SPROUTS WHERE POSSIBLE. I BRAISE OR STEAM MINE, OR ADD THEM TO STEWS AND SOUPS.

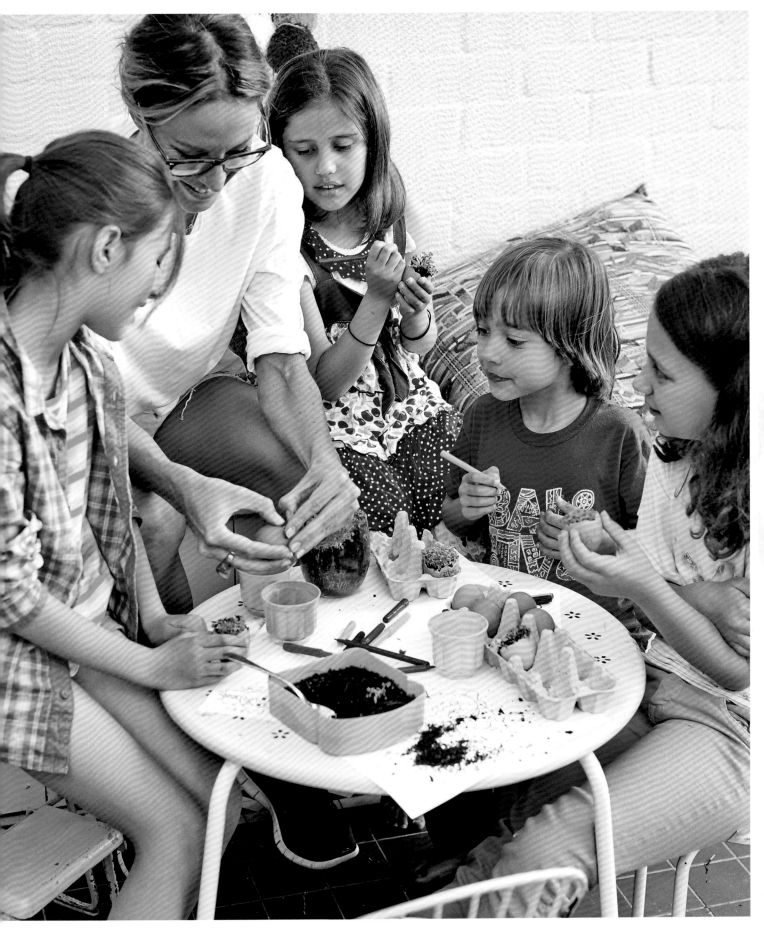

SPROUTED CHIA HEADS

Wash the empty eggshells thoroughly under warm running water, removing any membrane stuck to the inside. Fill with some soil and sprinkle the chia seeds on top of the soil. Spray thoroughly with water (you can use a garden hose) and leave for a day or two (not in direct sun), spraying the seeds lightly each day.

By day five or six the seeds will be ready to eat. Meanwhile, paint some eggcups with miniature outfits. Feel free to add limbs and other accoutrements. Give each one a name. Hey, look, Marija's sprouting!

Use old shoes, coffee mugs, dolls' heads that have the top cut off (actually this could be a little macabre!)...

chia seeds

empty eggshells

eggcups

acrylic paint

TIPS

FOR USING THE SPROUTS:

► Add to a peanut butter sandwich.

► Make Ants on a Log (see page 168).

► Toss through stir-fries, soups and salads.

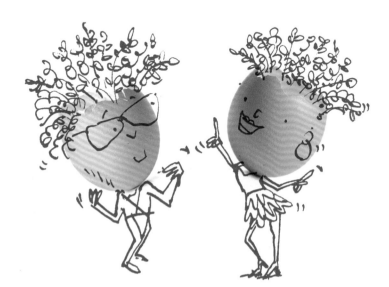

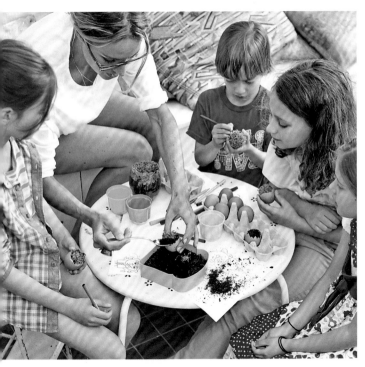
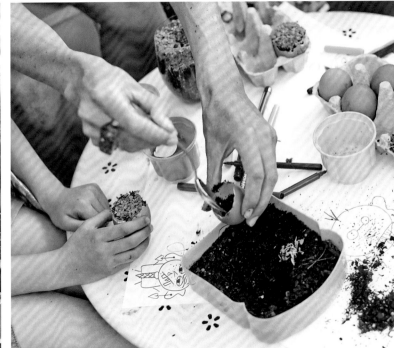
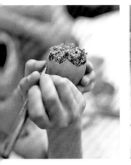
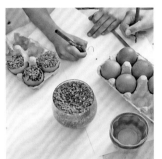
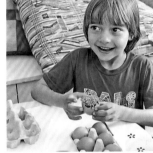
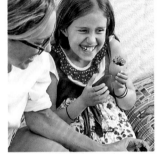
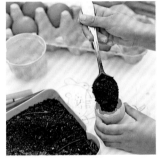
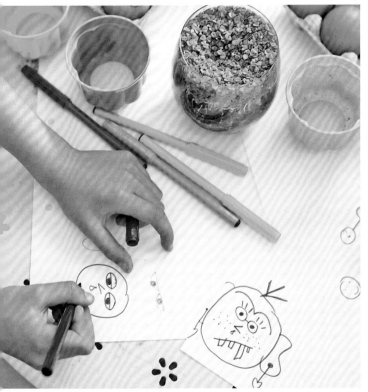
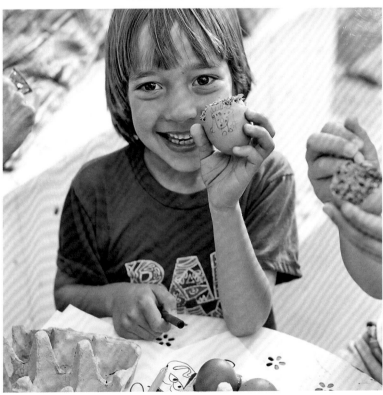

A WEEK of LUNCHBOX IDEAS

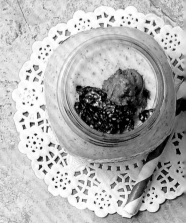

IT'S A FACT: kids' lunchboxes are little snap-shut vessels of horror when it comes to hidden (and not-so-hidden) sugar. A couple of commercial cereal bars together with a snack pack of sultanas adds up to about 22 teaspoons of sugar. Parents trying to do the right thing and follow guidelines are sickened to realise a standard muesli bar and a small apple juice 'popper' adds up to 12 teaspoons. And so mums and dads around the world collectively chorus, hands in the air: 'What are we meant to feed them?'

Here are a few ideas for the school lunchbox and afternoon tea snacks. Mix and match as you like, but try to sneak in as many vegetable items as possible.

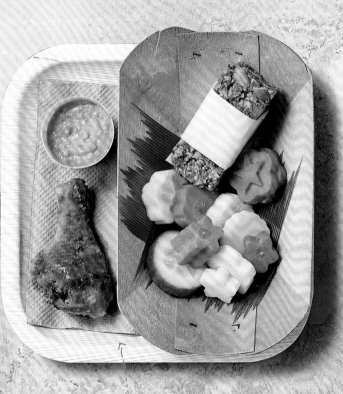

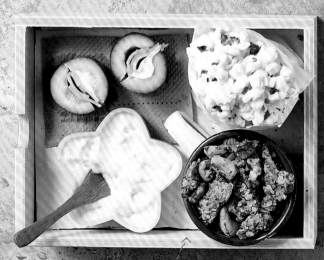

Monday

KFC DRUMSTICK (page 92) – call it a 'lollipop' and serve with a little container of Satay Sauce (page 207)

SPICED PUMPKIN GRANOLA BAR (page 156)

BENTO BITS (page 168)

Tuesday

CUCUMBER LAUGHING HEADS (page 168)

CHEESY 'GRAVY' (page 92)

POPCORN BAGS (page 168)

BOMBAY GRANOLA (page 158)

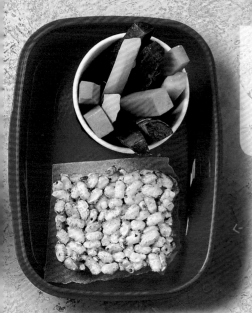

Wednesday

PEANUT BUTTER 'N' JELLY PORRIDGE WHIP (page 75)

COLOURED STICKS (orange and purple carrots and celery)

LCM BAR (page 152)

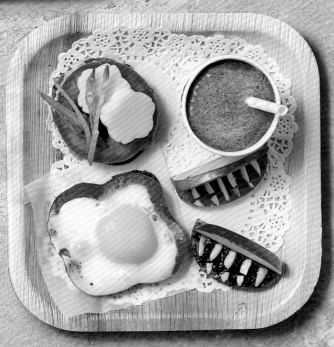

Friday

RAW BREAKFAST BALLS (page 68)

NOT-QUITE-APPLE-CRUMBLE MUFFIN (page 62)

ANTS ON A LOG (page 168)

LEFTOVER QUINOA MAC 'N' CHEESE (page 96)

[flick over for the recipes]

Thursday

SWEET POTATO BURGER (page 168)

GREEN SLIME SMOOTHIE (page 168)

FLOWER POWER EGGS (page 169)

NUTTY TEETH (page 168)

ANTS ON A LOG

Spread nut butter along a stick of celery and top with mung beans or other sprouts.

APPLE AND CHEESE SANDWICH

Spread Homemade Cream Cheese (see page 204, or the commercial stuff is fine) between two slices of apple.

BENTO BITS

Using a Bento cutter (you can buy these in speciality Japanese shops or online), cut cucumber, carrot, pepper, cheese, ham and cooked sweet potato slices into little shapes. Use the leftover bits in salads, casseroles and frittatas.

SWEET POTATO BURGERS

Bake sweet potato rounds coated in a little olive oil and salt in a 220°C (gas 7) oven for 20 minutes. Cool, then spread with avocado, a slice of tomato, cheese and mangetout cut into slivers.

CUCUMBER AND CHEESE SANDWICHES

Place a slice of cheese between two thick slices of cucumber. You could use a cookie cutter to cut the cheese into cucumber-sized rounds. Get the kids to do this with you the night before. They can stack them up to make 'triple burgers'.

NUTTY TEETH

Spread nut butter over a slice of apple and stick another slice into the nut butter at a 'jaw-like' angle. Spike some flaked almonds into both slices to form teeth.

CUCUMBER LAUGHING HEADS

Cut a cucumber in half lengthways and scoop out the seeds with a spoon. Fill one 'tunnel' with Homemade Cream Cheese (see page 204) and the other with a thinner layer of ham. Press the two layers together, then slice carefully into 3-cm rounds. Place two capers on the cream cheese layer for eyes.

PORRIDGE WHIPS [see pages 72 & 75]

These little packages combine two tricks. First, it's a no-cook porridge that's totally tote-able. Second, you soak the oats overnight, which makes them easier to digest.

POPCORN BAGS

Pour ¼ cup (50 g) of popcorn kernels into a brown paper bag and add a ½ tablespoon blob of coconut oil or butter. Shake and seal the bag by twisting it at the top. Microwave until there are 2 seconds between each pop.

GREEN SLIME SMOOTHIE

Blend 30 g of baby spinach leaves, 250 ml milk (any kind) and 150 g frozen strawberries with 1 frozen banana and ¼ cup (40 g) almonds soaked overnight in cold water (or almond meal) in a high powered blender until smooth and divide between 2 cups or jars.

TIP

Kids hate soggy tuna on sandwiches! To avoid this, mix the tuna with about 1 teaspoon of chia seeds. It becomes a thick 'spread' in about 5 minutes.

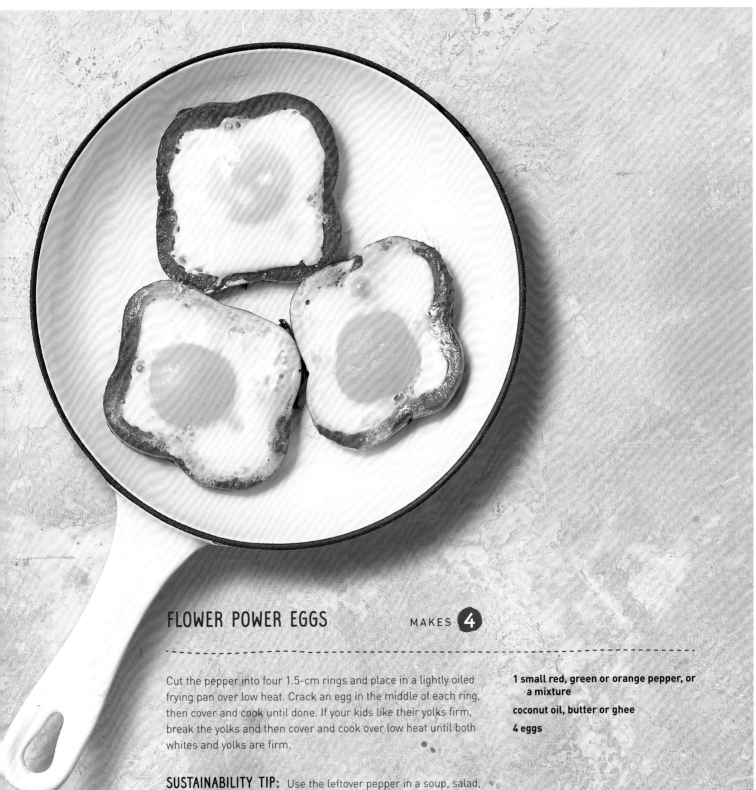

FLOWER POWER EGGS

MAKES **4**

- -

Cut the pepper into four 1.5-cm rings and place in a lightly oiled frying pan over low heat. Crack an egg in the middle of each ring, then cover and cook until done. If your kids like their yolks firm, break the yolks and then cover and cook over low heat until both whites and yolks are firm.

1 small red, green or orange pepper, or a mixture

coconut oil, butter or ghee

4 eggs

SUSTAINABILITY TIP: Use the leftover pepper in a soup, salad, juice, casserole or to make Bento Bits.

P **8WP** **CW**

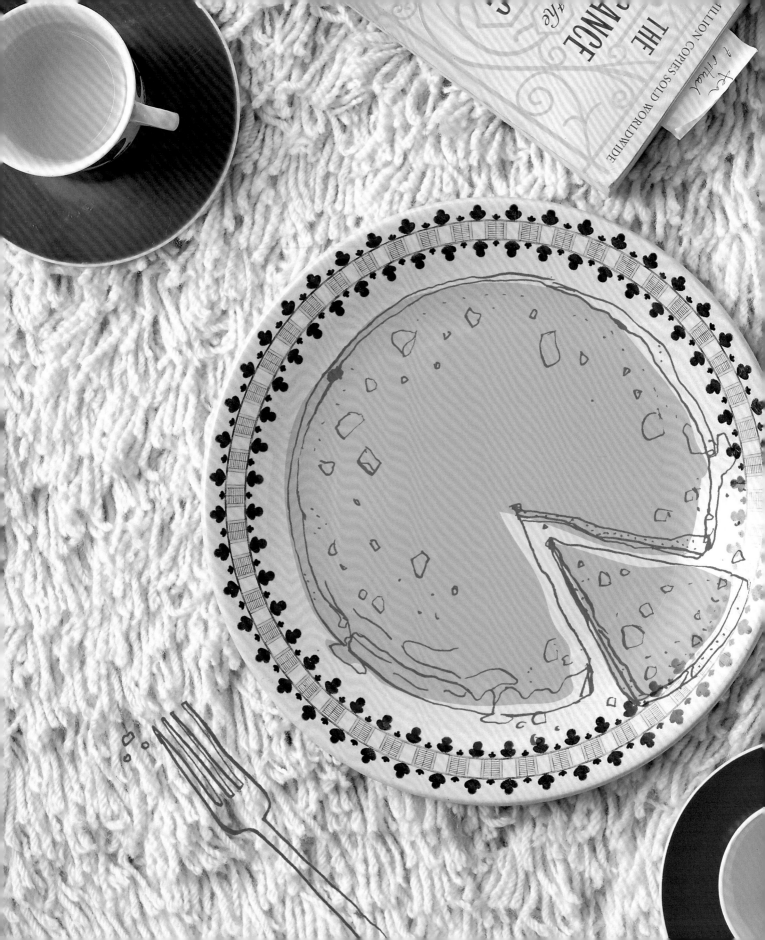

A CHAPTER OF CHOCOLATE

The recipes here are nutrient-dense
parcels of goodness.

Heck, some are healthy enough to eat
for breakfast (as I do!).

HANDMADE CHOCOLATE: Stuff you need to know

Chocolate can be a health food. I sometimes eat it for breakfast. True story. But it needs to be cooked and eaten the right way.

HOW TO EAT CHOCOLATE

1. RAW

When you read about those studies that report the amazing health benefits of chocolate, know this: they refer to raw cacao. Raw cacao powder is made by cold-pressing unroasted cocoa beans. The process keeps the living enzymes in the cocoa bean and removes the fat (cocoa butter). Cocoa powder is raw cacao that's been roasted at high temperatures. Sadly, roasting changes the molecular structure of the cocoa bean, reducing the enzyme content and lowering the overall nutritional value. If you're stuck, though, feel free to substitute cacao with cocoa 1:1.

2. WITH COCOA BUTTER NOT VEGETABLE OIL

Many commercial chocolates contain unhealthy poly-unsaturated oils, often palm oil, or PGPR. Why? Because it's cheaper than cocoa butter. Why should we care? Because these oils cause a lot of oxidative stress in our body and are linked to cancer and heart disease. Cocoa butter is the fat in cocoa beans that separates from the powder when the bean is cold-pressed (cacao) or roasted (cocoa). It's fantastic stuff. You can buy it in health food shops in buttons or chunks (that you'll need to grate before melting).

3. AS DARK AS POSSIBLE

A few recipes call for store-bought chocolate. If you're going to eat commercial chocolate, go for 85% cocoa varieties. A 70% variety is passable in small quantities. Do your maths and be aware of how much you're eating. Generally, whatever's not cocoa is sugar. So, a 70% cocoa chocolate bar will contain about 30% sugar. If you're eating a small 35 g bar, that's about 10.5 g sugar, or 2½ teaspoons. Be conscious of this.

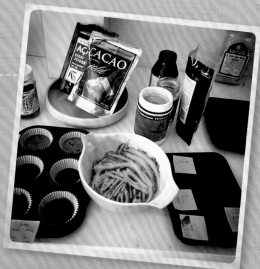

My experiments to find the perfect raw choc recipe.

IS CAROB OK? Short answer: No! It contains up to 50 per cent fructose, while the fructose content of cacao/cocoa is less than 1 per cent.

BEWARE

Most sugar-free chocolate is sweetened with maltitol, a sugar alcohol that passes straight to our large intestine, where it is broken down via fermentation by our gut bacteria, causing wind, bloating and diarrhoea. It has also been linked to the formation of cancer tumours.

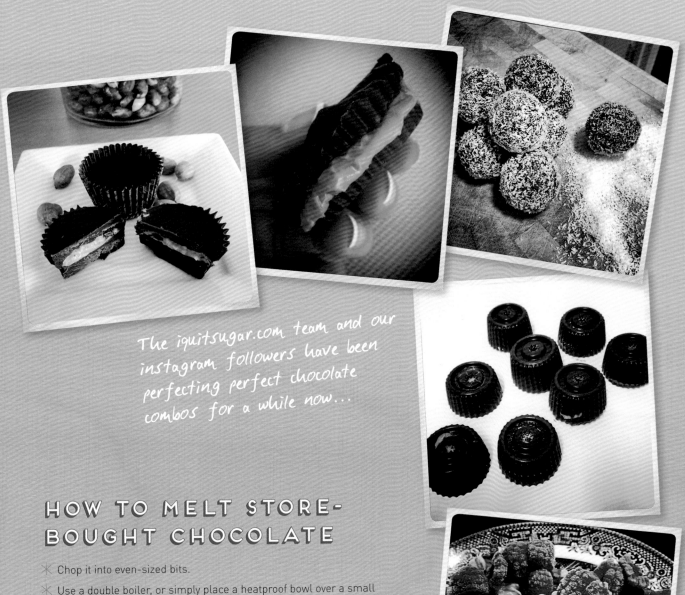

The iquitsugar.com team and our instagram followers have been perfecting perfect chocolate combos for a while now...

HOW TO MELT STORE-BOUGHT CHOCOLATE

✳ Chop it into even-sized bits.

✳ Use a double boiler, or simply place a heatproof bowl over a small saucepan with 2 cm of water in it.

✳ Simmer very gently over very low heat, stirring with a rubber spatula (never a wooden or metal spoon). (Chocolate retains its shape when melted, so the only way to know if it is actually melted is to stir it.)

✳ Stir continuously until your chocolate is shiny, smooth and completely melted.

✳ Chocolate melts faster than other liquids, so if you're also using milk, cream or coconut cream, melt these other liquids first. (This also helps prevent the chocolate from seizing.)

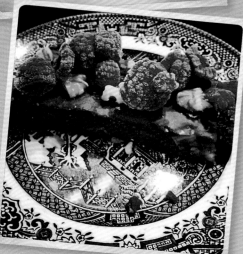

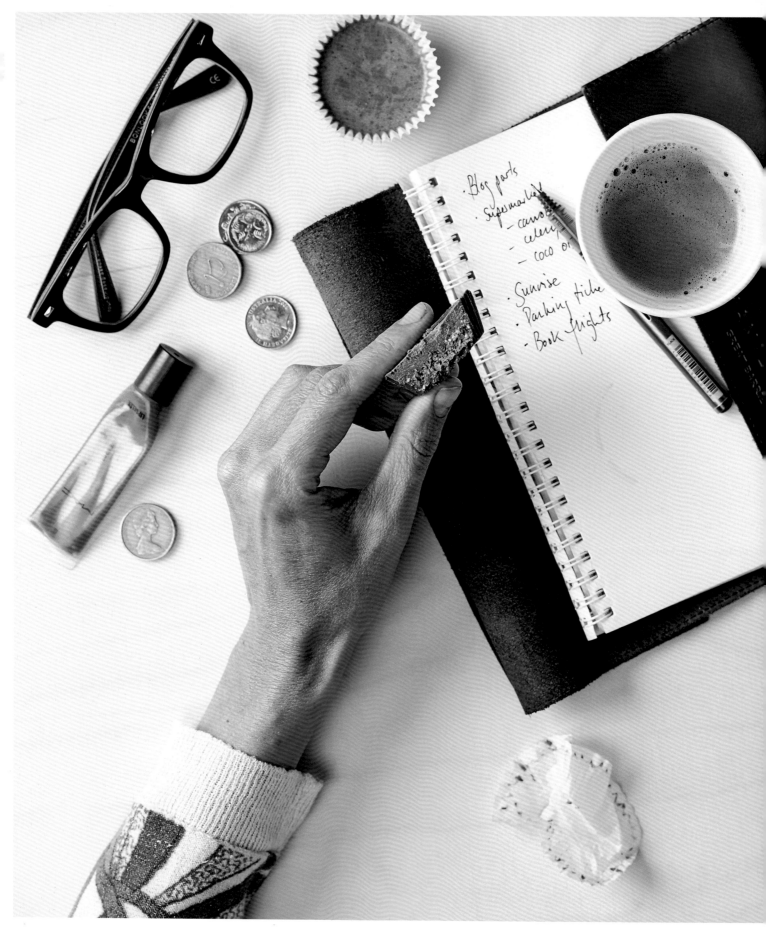

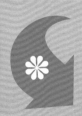

THREE WAYS with Raw Chocolate

BASIC RAW CHOCOLATE

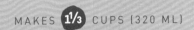

MAKES 1⅓ CUPS (320 ML)

I experimented with different ways of making chocolate for quite some time before arriving at what I believe to be the healthiest and 'sweetest' version. I then experimented and came up with the flavour bombs throughout this chapter.

Lightly grease some chocolate moulds or line a dinner plate with baking paper. In a small saucepan over low heat, melt the cocoa butter gently, stirring until smooth. Remove from the heat. Blend or mix with the rest of the ingredients until smooth and well combined. Add additional flavours if you like (see below), and stir. Pour into moulds or onto the prepared plate and freeze or refrigerate. Once hard, store in the fridge or freezer (raw chocolate melts at temperatures warmer than about 22°C). If you made your chocolate on the dinner plate, break into shards or 'bark', to serve.

- ½ cup (115 g) raw cocoa butter, buttons or shavings (if you don't have any, use an additional ½ cup (115 g) coconut oil instead)
- ½ cup (115 g) coconut oil, softened
- ⅓ cup (30 g) raw cacao powder
- 1–2 tablespoons rice malt syrup or 1–2 teaspoons granulated stevia
- 2 pinches of sea salt

1. FUDGY PROTEIN BITES

Throw 1⅓ cups (320 ml) melted Basic Raw Chocolate, ½–¾ cup (50–75 g) vanilla protein powder, ½ cup (75 g) chia seeds and ⅓ cup (40 g) maca powder (optional) or a little extra protein powder into a bowl to form a thick, pasty mixture. You may wish to add the protein powder and chia a little at a time, allowing the mixture to thicken slightly before adding more. Pour immediately into silicone moulds or cupcake cases and place in the fridge or freezer to harden. Makes 20–30.

2. CHOC CHILLI TRUFFLES

Combine 1⅓ cups (320 ml) melted Basic Raw Chocolate and 2 teaspoons ground cinnamon and 1 teaspoon cayenne pepper and pour immediately into silicone moulds or cupcake cases. Sprinkle with sea salt and place in the fridge or freezer to harden. Makes 20–30.

3. PEANUT BUTTER SHORTCAKES

These work best when the strawberries are pre-cut and frozen. Combine 1⅓ cups (320 ml) melted Basic Raw Chocolate and ½ cup (115 g) natural, sugar-free and salt-free peanut butter while the chocolate is still warm (so that the peanut butter can melt through). Stir through ½ cup (75 g) strawberries (cut into small pieces and pre-frozen if possible) and pour immediately into silicone moulds or cupcake cases. Makes 20–30.

ALMOST-PALEO COURGETTE BROWNIES

MAKES 16

Preheat the oven to 180°C (gas 4) and grease a 23-cm square brownie tin using the coconut oil, butter or ghee. Grate the courgettes into a large bowl, then add the rest of the ingredients and mix thoroughly. Pour into the prepared brownie tin and bake for 35 minutes or until a skewer comes out clean. Cool in the tin, then cut into squares.

NOTE: This recipe does contain quite a lot of intense, store-bought chocolate, which is why the serving sizes are quite small.

P

coconut oil, butter or ghee, for greasing

1 large or 1½ small courgettes

1 cup (225 g) almond (or any nut) butter

1 egg

½ teaspoon vanilla powder

4 tablespoons rice malt syrup

1 teaspoon ground cinnamon

¼ teaspoon ground nutmeg

1 teaspoon bicarbonate of soda

100 g dark (85% cocoa) chocolate, roughly chopped

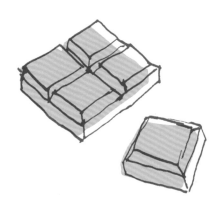

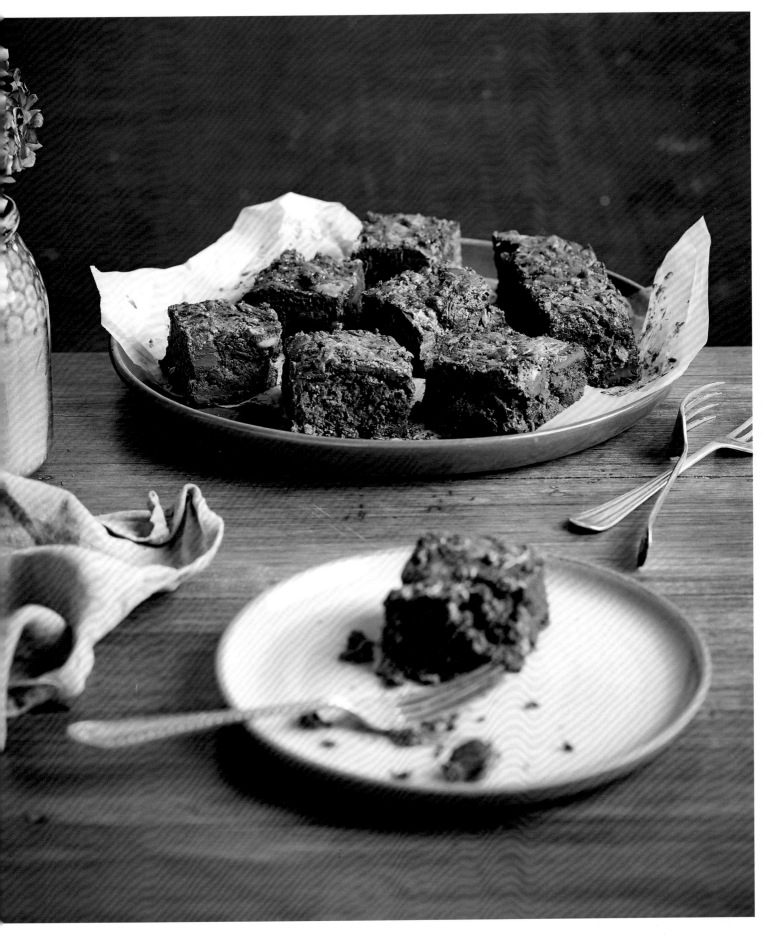

SWEET POTATO AND MACADAMIA FUDGE BROWNIES

Preheat the oven to 180°C (gas 4) and grease a 23 × 36-cm brownie tin using the coconut oil, butter or ghee. Put the Sweet Potato Purée in a bowl. Add the syrup, butter or oil, vanilla powder, flour, cacao powder, bicarbonate of soda, cayenne pepper and salt, and blend using a stick blender. Stir through the eggs, nuts and chocolate and pour into the prepared tin. Bake for 30 minutes or until cooked (see tip below). Allow to cool in the tin before cutting into squares.

WHAT'S YOUR TEXTURE?

I like my brownies a bit gooey. Test using a skewer; if it comes out a little moist, then you're good. If you like more of a cakey texture, cook for another 5–10 minutes. When the skewer comes out clean your brownies are ready.

This brownie is best when served cool and even better the next day!

coconut oil, butter or ghee, for greasing

1½ cups (350 ml) Sweet Potato Purée (see Pumpkin Purée variation on page 51)

⅓ cup (75 ml) rice malt syrup

90 g butter, softened, or ¼ cup (50 g) coconut oil

½ teaspoon vanilla powder

½ cup (50 g) self-raising flour (can be gluten-free)

⅓ cup (40 g) raw cacao powder

¼ teaspoon bicarbonate of soda

½ teaspoon cayenne pepper

pinch of sea salt

3 eggs, well beaten

¾ cup (175 g) roughly chopped macadamia nuts

½ cup (115 g) roughly chopped dark (85% cocoa) chocolate or cacao nibs

RAW CHOCOLATE STRAWBERRY BROWNIES

This one-pot wonder requires no baking! The recipe works better if you've chopped and frozen the strawberries in advance, but no drama if you only have fresh ones to hand.

Grease a 23 × 36-cm brownie tin using the coconut oil, butter or ghee. Blend all the ingredients except the strawberries and walnuts in a blender or using a stick blender. Stir in the strawberries and walnuts, pour into the prepared brownie tin and freeze for 1 hour. Cut into squares and store in the fridge.

coconut oil, butter or ghee, for greasing

⅓ cup (40 g) raw cacao powder

1 cup (100 g) almond or hazelnut meal

2 tablespoons chia seeds

1 cup (100 g) desiccated coconut

½ cup (125 ml) Pumpkin Purée (see page 51)

1 teaspoon vanilla powder (optional)

2 tablespoons coconut oil, melted

1 cup (150 g) strawberries, roughly chopped

2 cups (225 g) walnuts, roughly chopped

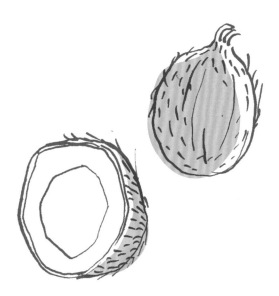

SIMPLE CHOCOLATE COCONUT MILK ICE CREAM

SERVES 4

Mix all the ingredients in a blender or using a stick blender until smooth and creamy. Pour into a freezer-safe container – a lunchbox will do – and leave in the freezer for 5 hours. (Or use an ice-cream maker, if you have one.) Serve with Ice Magic (see below) over the top. The ice cream may become a little too firm if left in the freezer too long. If so, allow it to thaw slightly before serving.

400 ml can full-fat coconut milk
⅓ cup (40 g) raw cacao powder
4 tablespoons rice malt syrup
½ teaspoon vanilla powder

ICE MAGIC

MAKES 1½ CUPS (350 ML)

Melt the coconut oil in a small saucepan over low heat then add the remaining ingredients, whisking well until the stevia is dissolved. Allow to cool slightly, then pour over homemade sugar-free ice cream. Store in a covered container in the fridge and melt when you need to use it.

½ cup (115 g) coconut oil
½ cup (50 g) raw cacao powder
¼ cup (50 g) granulated stevia
big pinch of sea salt

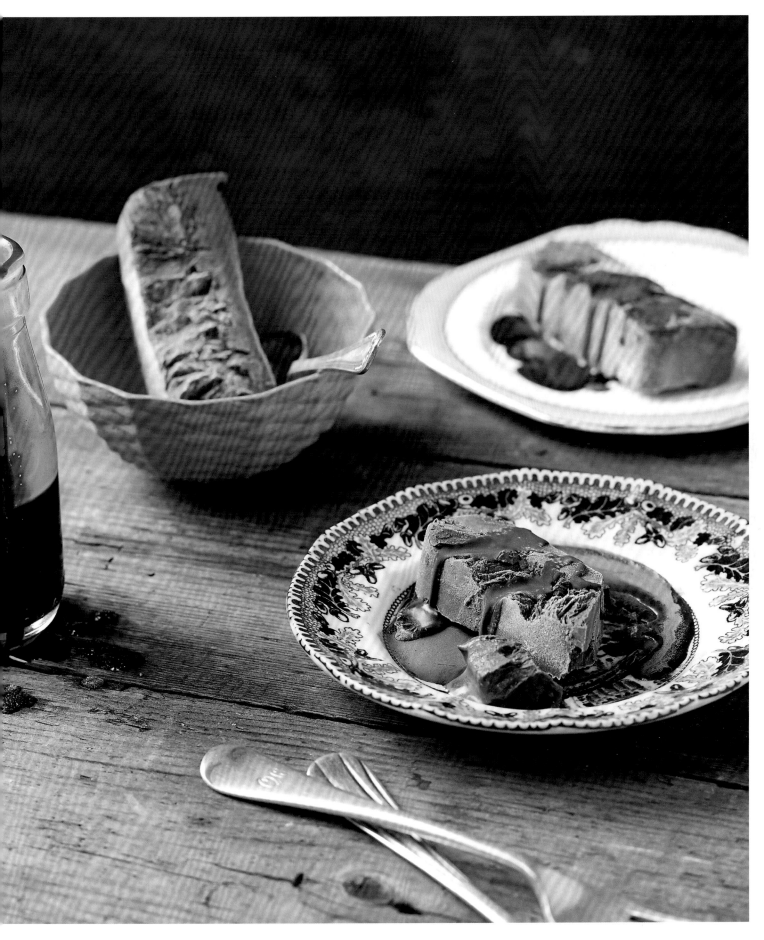

BEETROOT RED VELVET CUPCAKES

MAKES 12

Preheat the oven to 160°C (gas 3) and line a cupcake tin with 12 cupcake cases. Blend all the ingredients in a blender or using a stick blender to form a smooth batter, then pour into the cupcake cases. Bake for 40 minutes or until a skewer comes out clean. Serve alone or topped with yoghurt, Cream Cheese Frosting or Whipped Coconut Cream.

2 large beetroots, scrubbed, washed and grated (I personally don't bother peeling them)

2 eggs

½ teaspoon vanilla powder

1 teaspoon ground cinnamon

pinch of sea salt

1½ cups (150 g) almond meal

⅓ cup (40 g) raw cacao powder

4 tablespoons coconut oil or olive oil

4 tablespoons rice malt syrup

1 teaspoon baking powder

greek-style full-fat organic plain yoghurt, Cream Cheese Frosting (see below) or Whipped Coconut Cream (see page 72), to serve

CREAM CHEESE FROSTING

MAKES 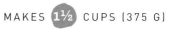 1½ CUPS (375 G)

Blend the cream cheese and butter in a blender or using a stick blender. Add the rest of the ingredients to blend, adding in extra lemon juice if it's too thick.

250 g Homemade Cream Cheese (see page 204, or you can use store-bought)

¼ cup (50 g) unsalted butter

4 tablespoons rice malt syrup or sugar-free icing mix

grated zest and juice of 1 lemon

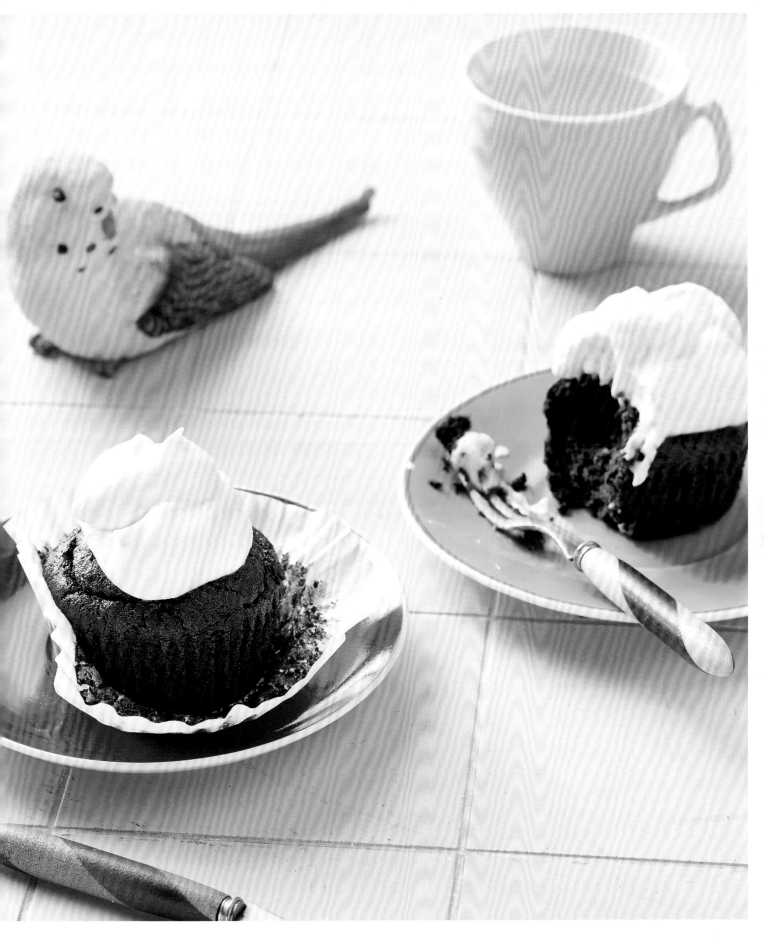

OH-OH OREOS

Preheat the oven to 180°C (gas 4) and line a baking tray with baking paper. Combine the flour, stevia and cacao in a large bowl or food processor. Add the diced cold butter and process or rub together using your fingertips until the mixture resembles fine breadcrumbs. Add the milk and syrup and mix to form a dough. Transfer to a lightly floured surface and knead for another minute or so, until the dough is nice and smooth.

Flatten the dough and place between two sheets of non-stick baking paper. Using a rolling pin, roll the dough out until it's about 4–5 mm thick. Cut out rounds and transfer to the prepared baking tray. Reroll the scraps and repeat the process. Prick each biscuit with a fork a few times. Bake in preheated oven for 10 minutes then transfer to a wire rack to cool.

To make the filling, whisk the cream cheese until light and creamy, then add the butter, rice malt syrup and vanilla powder and whisk until combined.

To assemble, place about 1 teaspoon of filling in the centre of half of the biscuits. Top with the remaining biscuits and squeeze together to push the filling to the edges.

Grown-up Variation:
MOCHA OREOS
Simply dissolve 2 teaspoons of instant coffee in the milk before adding to the crumb mix.

1 cup (115 g) gluten-free self-raising flour, plus extra for dusting

2 tablespoons granulated stevia

⅓ cup (40 g) raw cacao powder

75 g cold unsalted butter, diced

¼ cup (60 ml) milk

1 tablespoon rice malt syrup

FILLING

125 g Homemade Cream Cheese (see page 204), softened

25 g butter, softened

1 tablespoon rice malt syrup

½ teaspoon vanilla powder

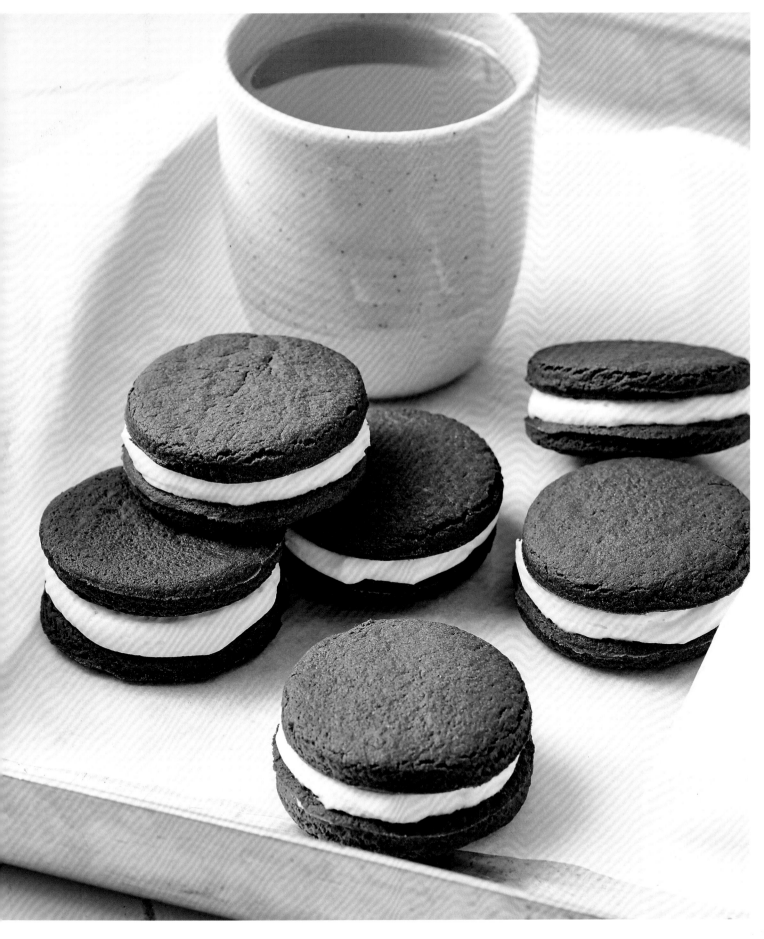

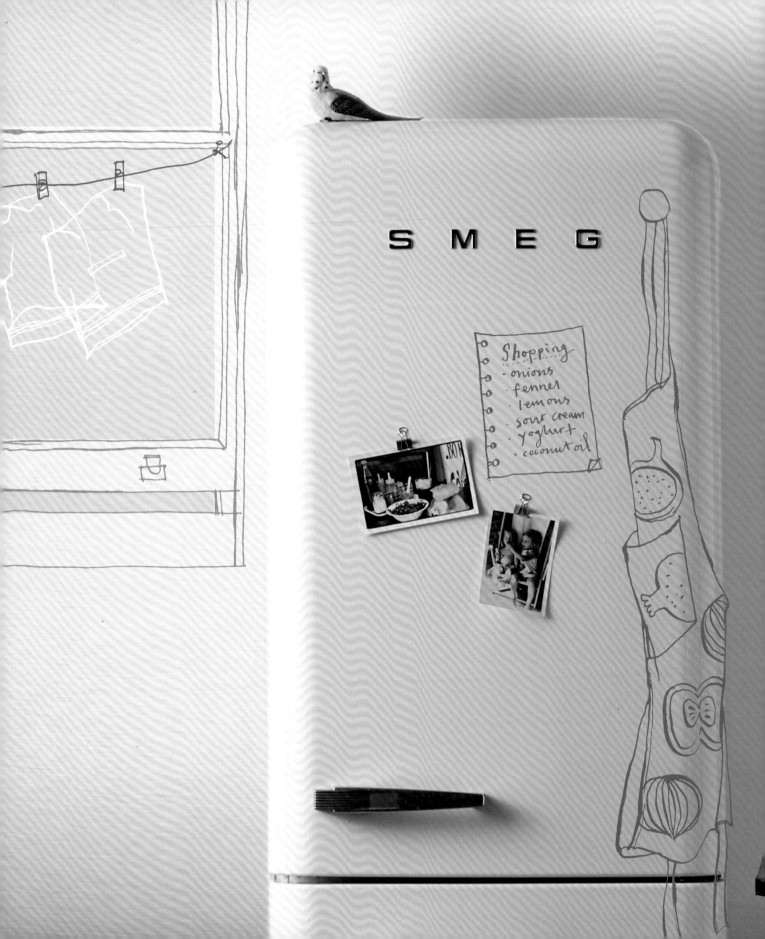

SMEG

Shopping
· onions
· fennel
· lemons
· sour cream
· yoghurt
· coconut oil

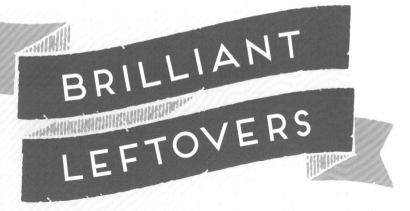

BRILLIANT LEFTOVERS

Food wastage kills me. If you're ever in a position
to need to impress me some day,
feed me your scraps, cook me up a
'fridge surprise' or repurpose.
last night's dinner.

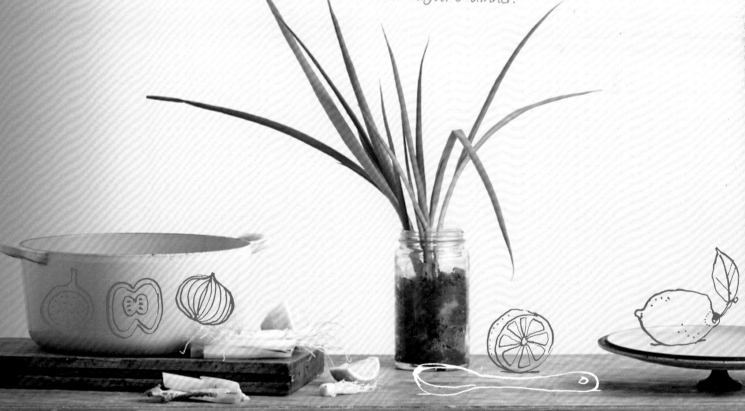

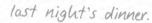

SWEET FENNEL AND BEETROOT LEAF SOUP

You know how you cooked up all those beetroots for the freezer (see page 51)?
Well, this is what you can do with the leaves.

In a large, stainless-steel saucepan over low heat, heat the butter or oil and gently and slowly cook the onion. Add the chilli, fennel or caraway seeds, fennel (not the fronds) and garlic, then cover and sweat until the fennel is soft, about 10 minutes. Add the beetroot leaves and stems, salt and pepper, lemon (as is; don't chop or squeeze) and stock. Bring to the boil, then turn off the heat immediately – the greens should be just wilted. Purée in the pan using a stick blender, or transfer to a blender in batches and blitz. Serve with a swirl of sour cream, yoghurt or cream cheese, garnished with the reserved fennel fronds.

NOTE: This soup is brilliant served cold, too.

2 tablespoons butter or olive oil

2 onions, sliced

¼ teaspoon chilli flakes

¼ teaspoon fennel seeds, crushed
(or caraway seeds, not crushed)

1 small bulb fennel, chopped,
green fronds reserved

2 cloves garlic, finely chopped

leaves and stems from 1 bunch of beetroots,
chopped

sea salt and freshly ground black pepper

½ lemon

5 cups (1.2 litres) Leftovers Chicken Stock
(see page 191)

½ cup (125 ml) sour cream, full-fat organic
plain yoghurt or 125 g Homemade Cream
Cheese (see page 204)

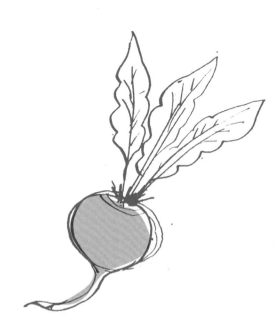

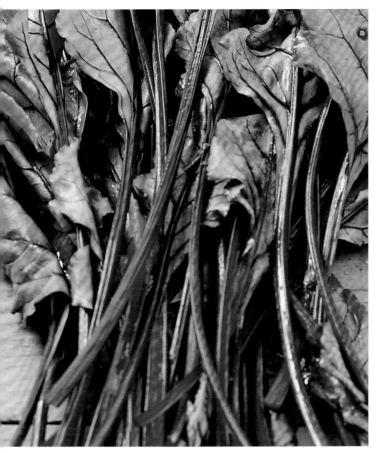

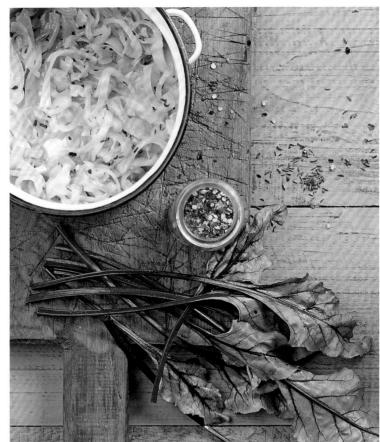

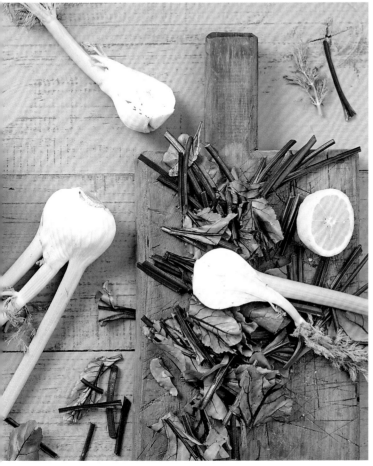

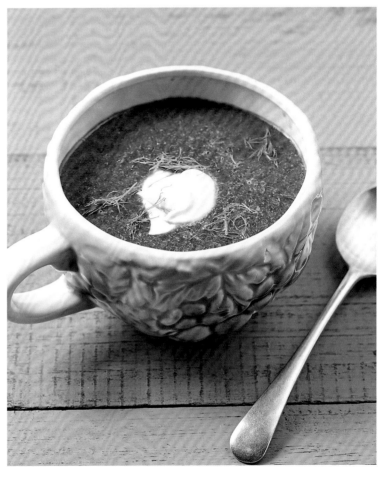

BONE BROTH

Bone broth is like normal stock but made with big, cheap bones you can get from your butcher (mine gives me them for free; yours will likely do the same or charge a minimal amount). The bones are simmered for a super loooong time (at least 12 hours), which leaches out a stack of minerals. These minerals are easy to digest in this soupy form and boost the immune system. Bone broth also contains glucosamine and chondroitin, which help those with arthritis and joint pain, and the gelatine is a boon for rebuilding the gut lining (hello, IBS sufferers!). And on and on go the benefits. I drink the stuff, warmed, when I'm run-down and feel the benefits immediately. It courses through my very being and I'm instantly energised.

Preheat the oven to 200°C (gas 6). Place the bonier bones (those with not much meat) in a very large stockpot with the vinegar and cover with cold water. Let stand for 1 hour. Meanwhile, put the meaty bones in a roasting pan and place in the oven until well browned. Add to the pot when they're ready, along with the vegetables.

Add additional water, if necessary, to cover the bones, but the liquid should come no higher than within 2.5 cm of the rim of the pot, as the volume expands slightly during cooking. The water should be cold – slow heating helps bring out the flavours. Bring to the boil. Reduce the heat and add the thyme and crushed peppercorns, then simmer for 12–72 hours.

When cool enough, use tongs or your hands to pull out the bones, then strain the rest into a large bowl. Refrigerate until cool and then, using tongs or large spoons, remove the layer of congealed fat on top – you can literally pick it up in chunks (like ice over a pond) – and toss it. Divide the remaining liquid into 1-cup (250 ml) portions and freeze for up to 6 months.

2–3 kg bones (beef marrow, knucklebones, meaty ribs, neck bones – whatever the butcher will give you)

½ cup (125 ml) white vinegar

2–3 onions, coarsely chopped

3 carrots, coarsely chopped

3 celery stalks, coarsely chopped

several sprigs of thyme, tied together

1 teaspoon dried green or black peppercorns, crushed

NIFTY FREEZING TIP

Here's a clever idea: freeze your stock in 1-cup (250 ml) jumbo muffin tins. Once frozen, pop them out and store in zip-lock bags labelled with the date ready to use in soups and dishes.

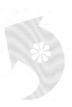

LEFTOVERS CHICKEN STOCK SERVES MAKES 1.5 LITRES

You can choose to make a chicken stock from scratch, picking out the meat to eat on its own (I included a recipe for my mum's chicken stock in my first book and you can also find this recipe on my blog, sarahwilson.com). Or you can do things the other way round – eat the meat first, then use the leftovers to good ends.

Place all the ingredients in a large stockpot with enough water to cover. Bring to the boil, then simmer, covered, for several hours – 2 is good, 3 is better, about 6 is best. When done, pull out the larger bits of chicken using tongs, then strain the stock into a container, discarding the bones and veggies. Place the stock in the fridge. After a few hours skim the fat off the top, then store the stock in the freezer in 1-cup (250 ml) batches or in ice-cube trays.

NOTE: The stock will keep for about 5 days in the fridge, longer if reboiled, and several months in the freezer.

1 chicken carcass, leftover from a roast dinner or any other whole chicken meal, including any bones people have chewed on (they're about to be boiled; don't fret about germs!)

1–2 cups (150–300 g) roughly chopped leftover offcuts of vegetables and herbs (carrots, celery, celery leaves, parsley, thyme)

3 bay leaves

sprinkle of peppercorns

splash of white vinegar

PUMPKIN PIKELETS

SERVES

Combine the Pumpkin Purée, flour, cinnamon and eggs in a small bowl. Heat some butter or oil in a small frying pan over medium heat and drop in 2-tablespoon dollops of the pikelet mixture. Cook for 3 minutes on each side, or until golden.

Serve with grated apple, walnuts, extra cinnamon, crumbled feta and a drizzle of rice malt syrup, or with crispy bacon and a dollop of yoghurt or a poached egg, or with Strawberry Jam (see page 207) and cream .

½ cup (125 ml) Pumpkin Purée (see page 51)

1 tablespoon plain flour

½ teaspoon ground cinnamon

2 eggs, lightly beaten

butter or coconut oil, for frying

SARDINIAN CELERY HEART SALAD   SERVES 4

Sardinia is another 'Blue Zone', boasting one of the highest number of centenarians in the world. Their diet, which contains little sugar, undoubtedly plays a role in their longevity. Sardinian cuisine also emerges from a history of poverty and, thus, the creative use of leftovers. How to live longer? Eat scraps! This is a modified version of a side dish I ate during a recent visit. It uses the base or heart of a bunch of celery, as well as the leaves, which are so often discarded.

Arrange the chicory or radicchio leaves in a serving bowl. Throw the celery heart, leaves, peas, chicory or radicchio stems and dressing into a separate bowl and toss well to combine. Arrange on top of the leaves and sprinkle with walnuts and cheese. Dress with Dressing in a Jar.

NOTE: If you can't find pecorino, use a soft goat's cheese, feta or shaved parmesan.

1 head chicory or small radicchio lettuce, leaves pulled apart, stem sliced very finely

1 celery heart, cut into even-sized pieces and very finely sliced

4 tablespoons celery leaves, chopped

¼ cup (40 g) frozen peas, thawed

¼ cup (25 g) roughly chopped walnuts

2 tablespoons shaved pecorino

2 tablespoons Dressing in a Jar (see page 205)

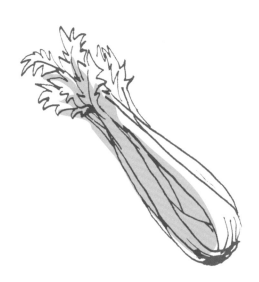

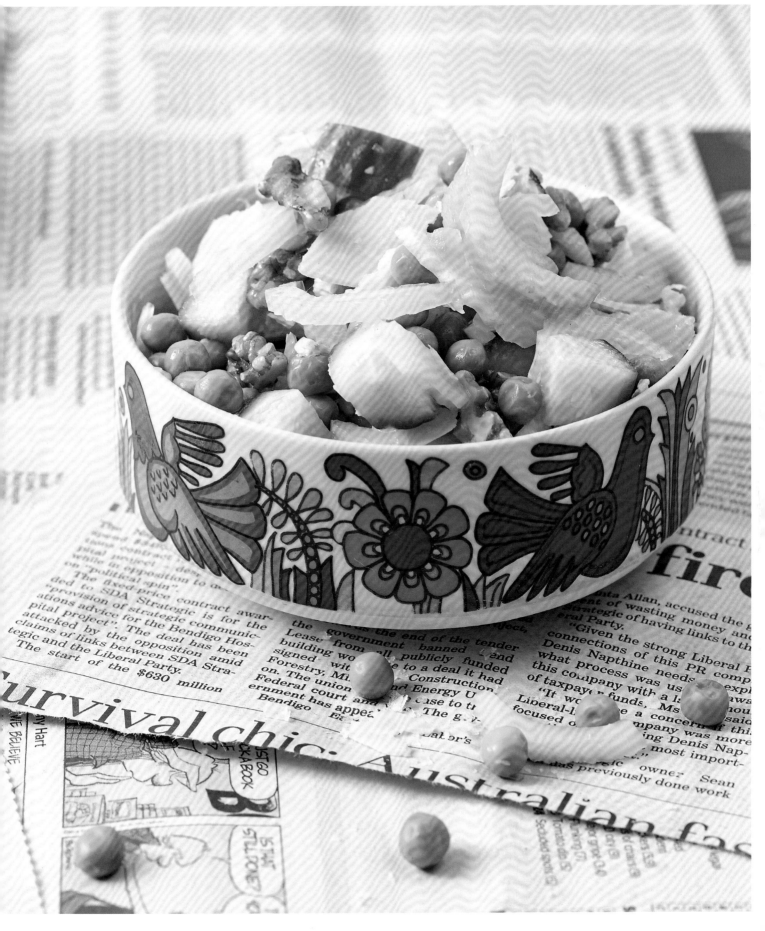

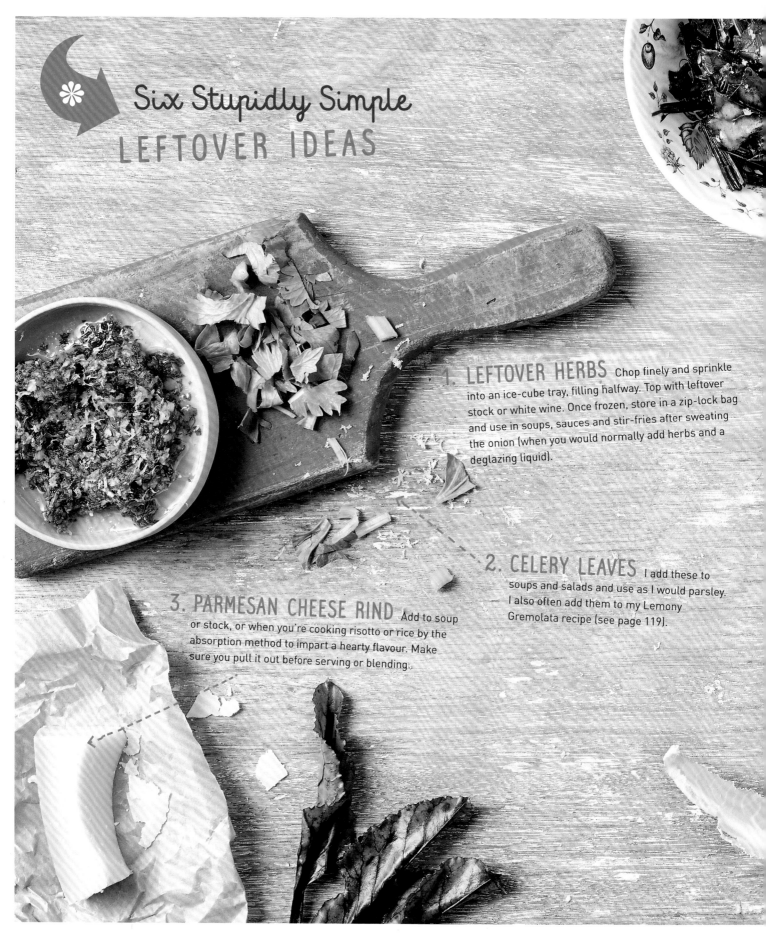

Six Stupidly Simple
LEFTOVER IDEAS

1. LEFTOVER HERBS Chop finely and sprinkle into an ice-cube tray, filling halfway. Top with leftover stock or white wine. Once frozen, store in a zip-lock bag and use in soups, sauces and stir-fries after sweating the onion (when you would normally add herbs and a deglazing liquid).

2. CELERY LEAVES I add these to soups and salads and use as I would parsley. I also often add them to my Lemony Gremolata recipe (see page 119).

3. PARMESAN CHEESE RIND Add to soup or stock, or when you're cooking risotto or rice by the absorption method to impart a hearty flavour. Make sure you pull it out before serving or blending.

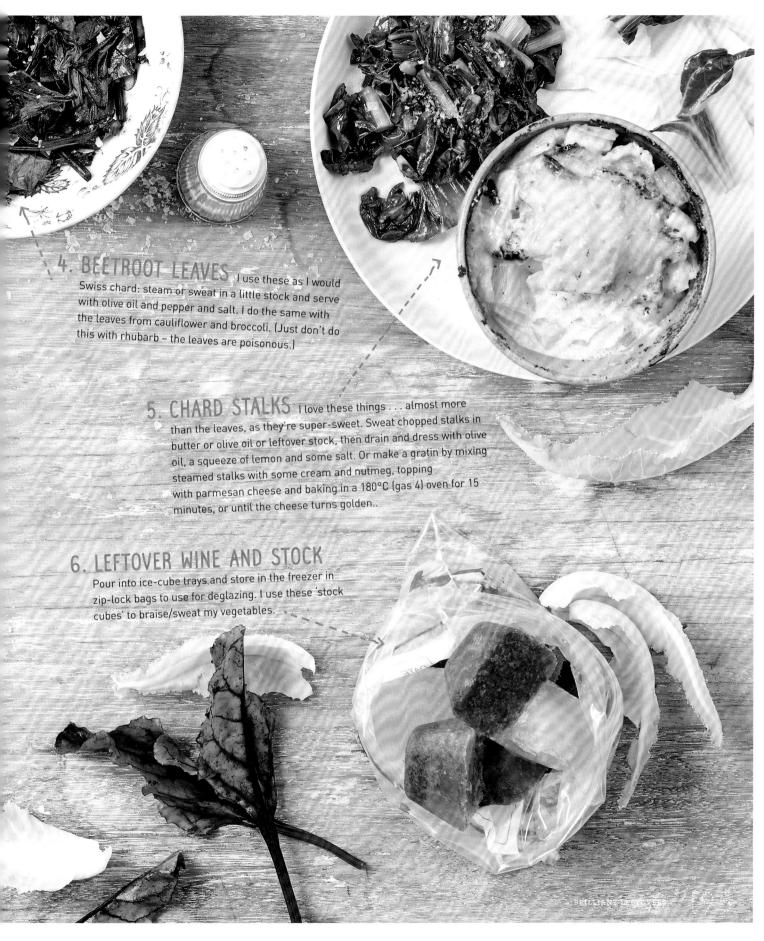

4. BEETROOT LEAVES
I use these as I would Swiss chard: steam or sweat in a little stock and serve with olive oil and pepper and salt. I do the same with the leaves from cauliflower and broccoli. (Just don't do this with rhubarb – the leaves are poisonous.)

5. CHARD STALKS
I love these things . . . almost more than the leaves, as they're super-sweet. Sweat chopped stalks in butter or olive oil or leftover stock, then drain and dress with olive oil, a squeeze of lemon and some salt. Or make a gratin by mixing steamed stalks with some cream and nutmeg, topping with parmesan cheese and baking in a 180°C (gas 4) oven for 15 minutes, or until the cheese turns golden..

6. LEFTOVER WINE AND STOCK
Pour into ice-cube trays and store in the freezer in zip-lock bags to use for deglazing. I use these 'stock cubes' to braise/sweat my vegetables.

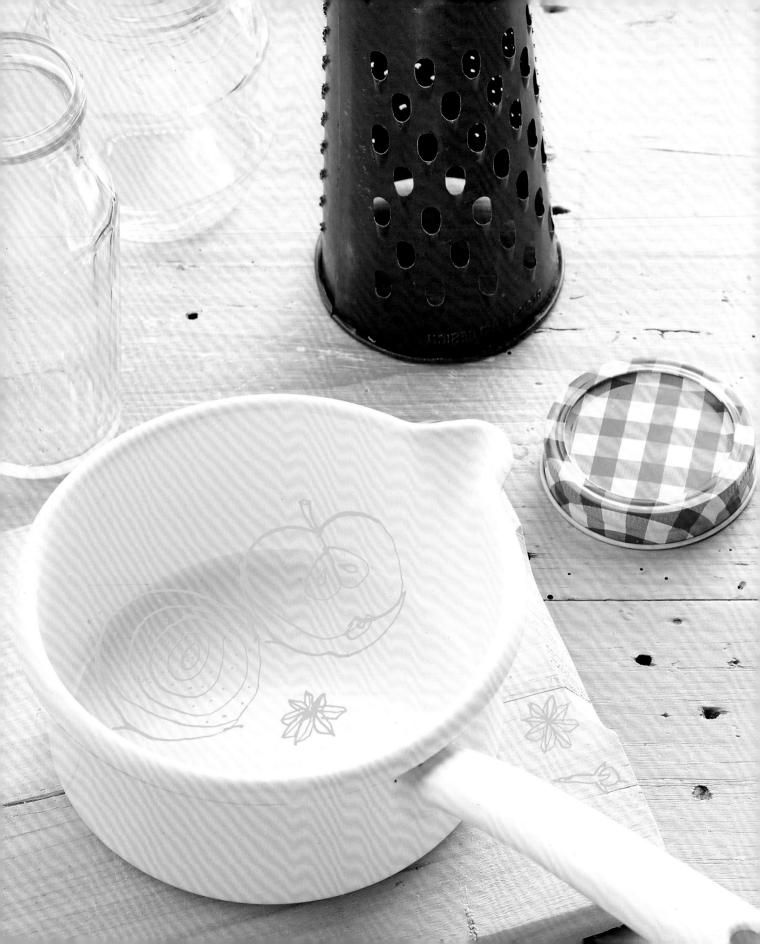

FERMENTS, SAUCES AND DRESSINGS IN JARS

All the things you need to add bursts of flavour to your cooking repertoire with the added bonus of being good for your guts.

Prepare a bunch of these — and their sister variations — and have them at the ready in your fridge.

I've designed them so they'll keep a while.

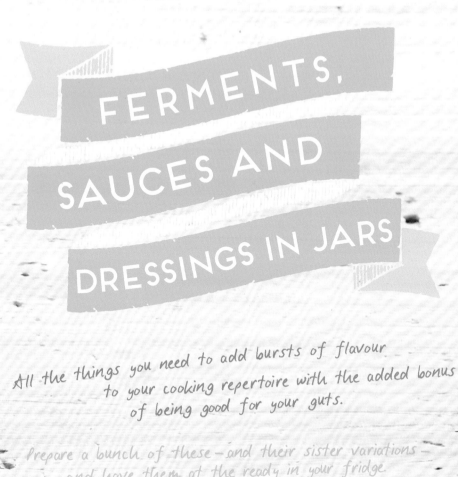

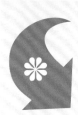

FOUR FABULOUS FERMENTS
for happier guts!

Countless cultures around the world have traditionally fermented their foods, in part as a preservation technique, but also as a way to enhance the nutritional profile of the ingredients.

Fermenting converts sugars – glucose, fructose and sucrose – into cellular energy and a metabolic by-product, lactic acid, which in turn produces fantastic digestive enzymes and healthy gut flora and cuts the sugar content of a food...all in one!

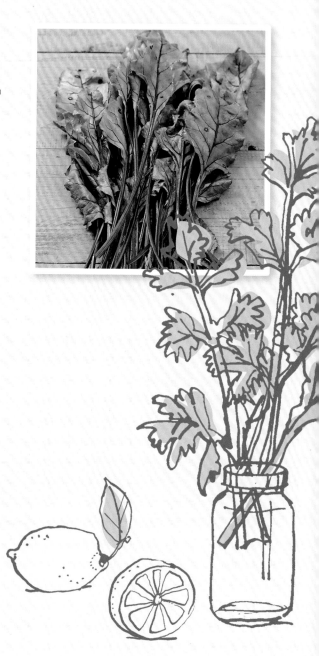

A FEW THINGS TO KNOW

▶ Use whey if you can – it works better. Whey is easy to make (see page 204) and can keep in the fridge for several weeks, in the freezer for months.

▶ Use super-fresh vegetables. Lactobacilli need plenty of nutrients to do their thing.

▶ Make sure you get a good centimetre of juices sitting above the veggies . . . otherwise mould grows, ruining the whole lot. That said, don't fret if your ferment gets bubbles or if little spots of white foam appear at the top of the liquid. This is totally normal and the spots can be lifted off with a spoon.

▶ If I don't extract enough liquid, I add a small amount of water with a pinch of salt dissolved in it.

▶ Don't open the jars while they're fermenting. The oxygen will spoil things.

▶ There's no need to sterilise jars and equipment. The 'local' bacteria are said to help the process.

▶ If you buy sauerkraut and kimchi in the shops, be aware many contain sugar and vinegar, and some are often pasteurised. All of which kills the lactic-acid-producing bacteria, which defeats the whole damn purpose.

1. BEETROOT and APPLE RELISH

Shred the apples and beetroot using a grater or a food processor. Toss together until well combined. Add the star anise and cloves, and continue to toss until the spices are evenly distributed. Spoon into a Mason jar a little at a time, periodically sprinkling salt and whey over each layer and mashing with a wooden spoon or mallet so the juices are released. Leave to ferment at room temperature for 3–4 days.

Pick out the star anise and cloves and discard them. Blend the relish in a food processor or using a stick blender until smooth.

3 large apples, cored but not peeled

4 large beetroots, peeled

2 star anise

1 tablespoon cloves

¾ tablespoon sea salt

**4 tablespoons whey (see page 204), optional
  or an extra 1 teaspoon salt**

---

2. FERMENTED Cucumbers

MAKES **2** – **3** CUPS (500–750 ML)

These are like pickled cucumbers, which are made using sugar and/or vinegar. Look for pickling or ridge cucumbers. Regular cucumbers will do almost as well, but you'll need to ensure they're as fresh as possible, with a tight, firm skin.

Choose a wide-mouthed jar tall enough to fit the cucumbers with 3 cm to spare. Wash the cucumbers, chop 1 cm off both ends and submerge them in iced water for an hour. Put the cucumbers in your chosen jar; leave whole or cut into spears if you're struggling to get them to fit. Place the dill, garlic, fennel seeds and peppercorns in the jar. Combine the salt, whey and water, stirring to dissolve the salt, then pour into the jar (topping with extra water if necessary to cover the cucumbers). The cucumbers will float as they ferment, so place a small ramekin or saucer on top. Put on the lid and keep at room temperature (preferably 18–21°C – whack it in a cool laundry or bathroom if required) for about 3 days (longer if you like them sour) before transferring to the fridge. They will last about 1 month before they go soft.

**6 pickling cucumbers
  (or 5 small, firm regular cucumbers)**

4 dill fronds

**2 cloves garlic, peeled and smashed with
  the back of a knife**

½ teaspoon fennel seeds, lightly smashed

1 teaspoon peppercorns

1 tablespoon sea salt

5 tablespoons whey (see page 204)

1½ cups (350 ml) water

3. HOMEMADE Sauerkraut

MAKES **3** — **4** CUPS (750 ML–1 LITRE)

Mix all the ingredients in a sturdy bowl and pound with a wooden mallet or meat hammer, or just squeeze with your hands (this is actually very soothing and meditative), for about 10 minutes to release the juices. This takes a little work and some patience. Spoon into a Mason jar and, using the pounder or meat hammer, press down until the juices come to the top of the cabbage and cover it. Cover tightly and keep at room temperature for about 3 days before transferring to the fridge where it will keep for several months.

1 medium cabbage, cored and shredded

1 tablespoon caraway seeds

1 tablespoon sea salt

5 tablespoons whey (see page 204) or an extra 1 tablespoon salt

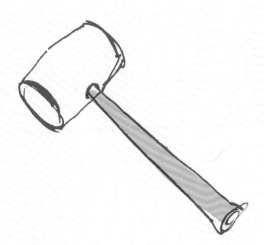

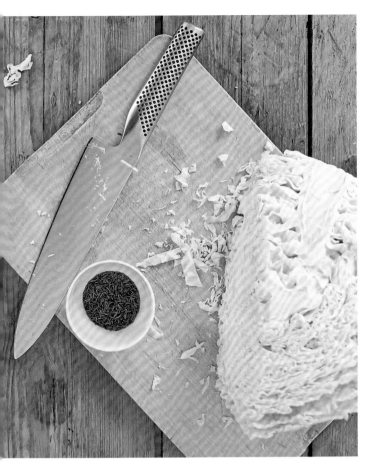
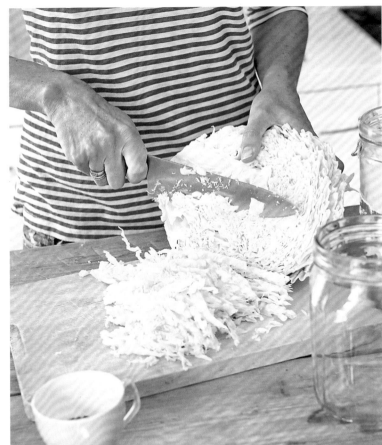
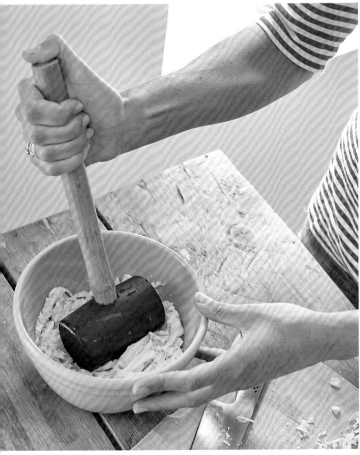
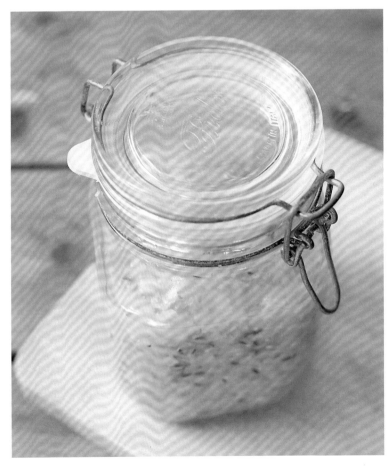

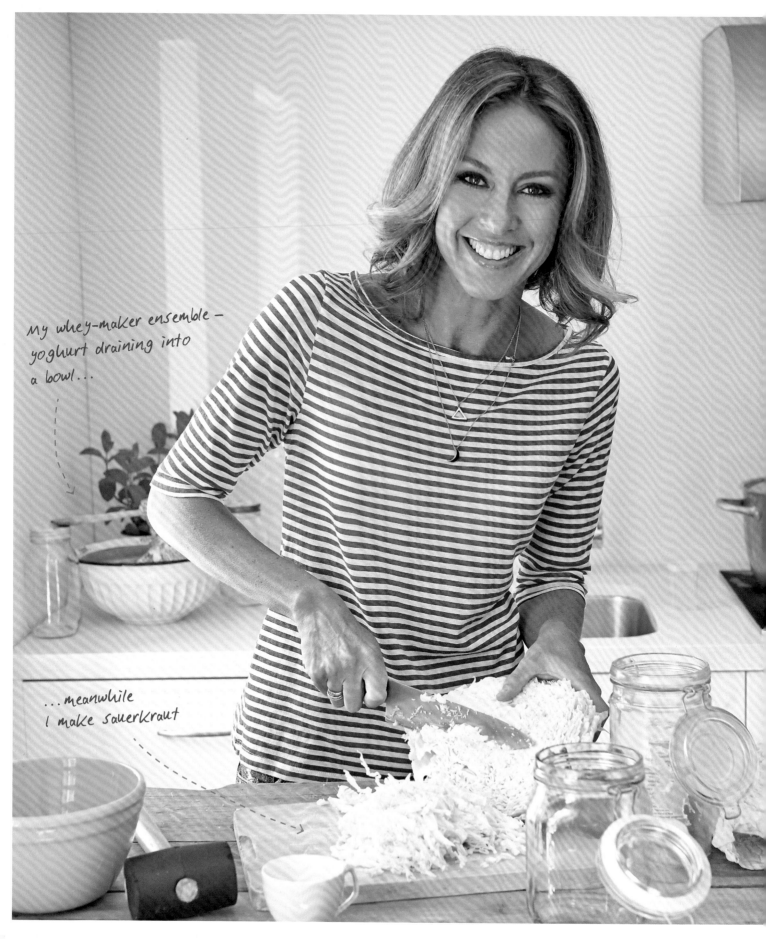

My whey-maker ensemble —
yoghurt draining into
a bowl...

...meanwhile
I make sauerkraut

4. GINGERADE

 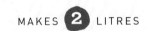

Table sugar – yes! – is almost always used for making fermented sodas, but the fructose is 'eaten up' in the process by yeast and bacteria, to create lactic acid and carbonation. Lactic acid is a probiotic that helps digestion, supports the immune system and hydrates cells.

Now, I was a little dubious about whether all of the sugar is used up in this process and did a lot of research into the matter. It seems that, after a 48-hour fermentation period, 80 per cent of the sugar has been gobbled up by the yeast and bacteria. Extrapolated, this means 25 g sugar is left in 2 litres of my gingerade. In 1 cup (250 ml) of the stuff, it's 3.1 g sugar, which is about ¾ teaspoon. If consumed with soda water (I find it works best half gingerade, half soda), then one large glass will contain less than ½ teaspoon sugar.

To cut things back further I tried out versions using a combo of sugar and rice malt syrup. Feel free to use no sugar at all and use a total of ¾ cup (180 ml) of rice malt syrup instead. But bear in mind it will require a slightly longer fermentation period. All good. This recipe is the base for my Yule Mule Cocktail. Check it out, page 146.

Pour the water into a saucepan, then mix the sugar and syrup together and stir into the water. Bring to the boil and simmer for 10 minutes. Cool to room temperature, then add the ginger, lemon zest and juice. (If you have a high-powered blender, trim the zest off the lemons and blitz, then trim away the pith and discard, along with any visible pips, then add the lemon flesh to the blender and blitz again.) Transfer to a Mason jar and add the whey.

Stir well and leave to sit on the worktop, stirring occasionally, for 2–3 days in hot weather, longer in cooler climates, or until slightly bubbly and becoming tart. Strain the gingerade into bottles. Allow to carbonate for another 2–3 days at room temperature, chill, then consume. If you're not going to drink it straight away, keep it in the fridge – it will keep fermenting, even in the cold, and last a week in the fridge before it goes vinegary. The longer it's left to ferment, the tangier it will get.

NOTE: I tend to drink this 1:1 with soda water. This adds extra fizz and spreads the goodness further.

6 cups (1.5 litres) water
½ cup (115 g) sugar
4 tablespoons rice malt syrup
1 cup (100 g) thinly sliced unpeeled fresh ginger
grated zest and juice of 2 lemons
½ cup (125 ml) whey (see page 204)

HOMEMADE CREAM CHEESE

MAKES **1** CUP (250 G)

Pour the whole tub of yoghurt onto a large handkerchief-sized square of clean cheesecloth or muslin. Bunch the ends like you're tying a sack and secure with an elastic band or string. Suspend the bag over a large bowl – I attach mine to a wooden spoon placed across a bowl, while others hang theirs from a cupboard doorknob, or even a chandelier! You're going to be straining out the whey, leaving a beautifully creamy curd in the sack. Drain for 12–24 hours.

Store the cream cheese in the fridge for up to 1 month. Keep the whey (it will keep in the fridge for 3 months or you can store it in batches in the freezer) for fermenting vegetables (to make them last longer, see page 198) or making mayonnaise (see page 208).

NOTE: Whey is used in many recipes in this book so look out for cross references.

1 kg tub full-fat organic plain yoghurt

ORGANIC ALERT

Be sure to use full-fat *organic* plain yoghurt – I've found that this recipe doesn't work well if you use the more commercial stuff.

ACTIVATED NUTS

I know, I know. Many gags have been made about these things of late. But entendres aside, nuts that have been activated really are worthwhile contributions to the food chain. Nuts and seeds contain poisons in the husk that can make them tough to digest. Soaking then drying them causes them to sprout, which activates enzymes that make them easier to digest and metabolise. Activating also produces a crunchier, slightly toasty version of the original nut or seed. Almonds, walnuts, pistachios, pecans and pumpkin seeds work best – the 'oily' nuts such as macadamias or cashews can go a little soggy, and must be soaked for no longer than 6 hours.

Soak the nuts or seeds overnight in a covered saucepan of water with the salt. Drain, then spread out on a baking tray (no oil, no baking paper) and dry in the oven for 12–24 hours at the lowest temperature possible (less than 65°C for gas ovens, on the pilot light). When cool, store in a sealed container in the freezer.

1 x bag of non-oily nuts or seeds (e.g. almonds, pumpkin seeds, walnuts)

pinch of sea salt

water

STORING YA NUTS

Store your nuts in the freezer – they keep fresher for longer and are crunchier! Plus you can eat them straight from the freezer, as they don't actually freeze.

DRESSING IN A JAR

MAKES ¾ CUP (180 ML)

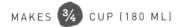

¼ cup (60 ml) apple cider vinegar
½ cup (125 ml) olive oil
½ teaspoon rice malt syrup
big grind of sea salt and black pepper

Place all the ingredients in a jar and shake vigorously.

1. A-LITTLE-BIT-FRENCHY DRESSING

Make the Dressing in a Jar but add 1 tablespoon Dijon mustard.

2. TAKE-ME-ANYWHERE ASIAN DRESSING

Make the Dressing in a Jar (you can use rice vinegar instead of apple cider vinegar). Add 1 tablespoon of soy sauce or tamari, 1 tablespoon of sesame seeds, 2 teaspoons of grated fresh ginger and 1 teaspoon of sesame oil. Shake vigorously.

3. ALKALISING POTION

This dressing is a detox juice used as a dressing. Pour it liberally over salads, meat and vegetables when sugar cravings or lapses hit. Make the Dressing in a Jar. Add 2 tablespoons of lime juice, 2 tablespoons of chopped fresh coriander and ¼ teaspoon of cayenne pepper. Shake vigorously.

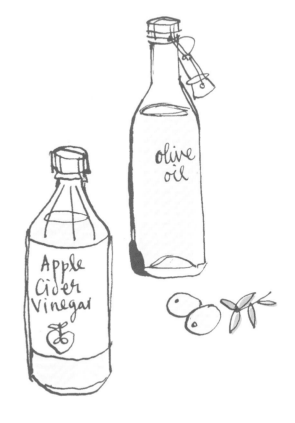

BETTER THAN A BOTTLE *everyday sauces*

HOMEMADE TOMATO SAUCE

Commercial tomato sauce is often up to 45 per cent sugar. My version does contain a lot of tomatoes (and generally I steer my choices away from concentrated tomato-based stuff as they use up so much of the fruit: the fructose adds up), but if you're eating it as a condiment – only a tablespoon or two – you're right as rain.

Bring all the ingredients to the boil in a saucepan, stirring to distribute the spices. Reduce the heat and simmer for about 50 minutes or until the sauce reduces by almost half and is quite thick. Blend with a stick blender or in a food processor. If the sauce is still a bit runny, return it to the heat and reduce for a little longer. Store in a clean glass jar in the fridge for up to 1 month. (I divide my mixture and freeze half so it doesn't spoil.)

NOTE: You can also do this in an electric slow cooker: cook all the ingredients on high for 2–2½ hours. After blending, you might want to return it to the cooker for another 30 minutes, without the lid, to thicken.

Homemade BBQ Sauce Variation:

Mix together 250 ml Homemade Tomato Sauce, 2 tablespoons apple cider vinegar, 1 teaspoon Tabasco sauce, 1 clove garlic (finely chopped), 1 tablespoon paprika and 2 tablespoons chilli powder. Makes about 300 ml. Keeps in the fridge for up to 1 month.

TERIYAKI SAUCE

Make as for the Take-Me-Anywhere Asian Dressing (see page 205) but omit the olive oil and the sesame seeds, and triple the soy sauce or tamari and the sesame oil.

2 × 440 g cans whole peeled tomatoes or 675 ml passata

½ onion, chopped

⅓ cup (75 ml) apple cider vinegar

1 tablespoon rice malt syrup (or 2 teaspoons granulated stevia)

1 teaspoon ground allspice

1 teaspoon ground cinnamon

1 teaspoon ground cloves

1 teaspoon cayenne pepper

sea salt and freshly ground black pepper

I QUIT SUGAR FOR LIFE

DECEPTIVELY SWEET CHILLI SAUCE

MAKES 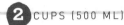 CUP (150 ML)

The commercial stuff is generally a very gooby affair, achieved through large amounts of sugar, rendering it more sugary than ice-cream topping. True story.

Purée the vinegar, stevia, chillies, water, fish sauce, garlic and salt in a blender, or finely chop the chilli and garlic first then combine with the rest of the ingredients in a jar, shaking vigorously. Pour the mixture into a saucepan and bring to the boil. Reduce the heat and simmer for 5–10 minutes until reduced by about half. Meanwhile, combine the cornflour or arrowroot and 2 tablespoons of extra water to make a thick paste. Whisk the paste into the sauce and simmer for 1 minute more. Cool and store in a glass jar in the fridge for 1 month.

½ cup (125 ml) rice vinegar or apple cider vinegar

¼ cup (50 g) granulated stevia

2 red chillies (deseed if you don't like your sauce too hot) or ½–1 tablespoon chilli flakes

¼ cup (60 ml) water

¼ cup (60 ml) fish sauce

3 cloves garlic

½ teaspoon sea salt

1 tablespoon cornflour or arrowroot

2 tablespoons water (extra)

SATAY SAUCE

MAKES ABOUT 2 CUPS (500 ML)

Throw all the ingredients into a small saucepan and bring to the boil over medium heat. Reduce the heat to low and cook for 10 minutes, stirring occasionally, for the sauce to thicken. Transfer to a jar and keep in the fridge for 2–3 weeks.

400 ml can coconut cream

½ cup (115 g) natural, sugar-free and salt-free crunchy peanut butter

1 teaspoon ground turmeric

1 teaspoon ground ginger

1 teaspoon ground coriander

pinch of ground cumin

½ teaspoon sea salt

STRAWBERRY JAM

MAKES ABOUT 2 CUPS (500 ML)

Throw all the ingredients into a blender and blend until smooth, then pour into a saucepan and heat over medium heat until the mixture begins to bubble. Reduce the heat and whisk constantly until thickened, about 3–5 minutes.

1 cup (150 g) strawberries (frozen or fresh)

1 cup (250 ml) water

2 tablespoons rice malt syrup

2 tablespoons chia seeds or arrowroot

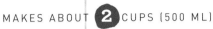

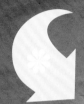

Five Ways with...

WHEY-GOOD MAYO

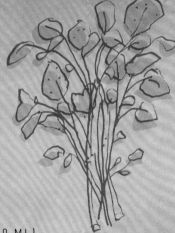

HAVE YOU MADE YOUR OWN MAYO YET? It's one of those kitchen staples that is so Martha-Stewart-y satisfying to make. Apron pinned, you really feel like you've completed a worthwhile, homely project. I make mine with whey. Why? It turns the condiment into an activated, stomach-benefiting food, plus it means it will keep for 3 months instead of 2 weeks. I make a batch then divide it up and choose my own adventure with a bunch of different flavours.

WHEY-GOOD MAYO

MAKES **1½** CUPS (350 ML)

Whizz all the ingredients except the oil in a food processer on a low speed for 30 seconds. With the motor running (still on low), very slowly drizzle in the oil until the mayo is thick and smooth. (Did I mention to drizzle it very slowly? You want it to pour in a very, very fine stream, otherwise it won't form an emulsion.) If you included the whey, cover the mayonnaise and let it sit at room temperature for 8 hours before refrigerating. This activates the enzymes in the whey. If you didn't use whey, refrigerate immediately.

1 egg
1 teaspoon Dijon mustard
1 tablespoon lemon juice
1 tablespoon whey (see page 204, optional)
big pinch of sea salt
1 cup (250 ml) extra-virgin olive oil

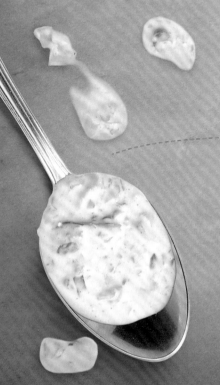

1. TARTARE SAUCE

MAKES **¾** CUP (180 ML)

1 tablespoon chopped Fermented Cucumbers
    (see page 199, optional)
½ tablespoon capers
1 tablespoon spring onions
juice of ½ lemon
½ cup (125 ml) Whey-Good Mayo
pinch each of sea salt, freshly ground black pepper
    and cayenne pepper

Pulse the fermented cucumber, capers and spring onions in a blender or food processor (not too fine; you don't want a purée). Add the lemon juice, mayo and seasoning, and stir.

NOTE: You can get extra greenery into this by adding ¼ leftover lettuce (gem or cos).

2. THOUSAND ISLAND DRESSING MAKES CUP (125 ML)

½ cup (125 ml) Whey-Good Mayo
½ tablespoon rice malt syrup
1 tablespoon harissa paste
sea salt and freshly ground black pepper
juice of ½ lemon

Whisk or blend all the ingredients together.

3. KOREAN MAYO MAKES CUP (185 ML)

½ cup (125 ml) Whey-Good Mayo
4 tablespoons Take-Me-Anywhere Asian Dressing
  (see page 205)
½ teaspoon chilli flakes

Combine all ingredients and whisk or blend.

NOTE: You can also make this by simply
combining the Whey-Good Mayo with 4
tablespoons Take-Me-Anywhere Asian Dressing
and adding ½ teaspoon crushed dried chilli flakes.

4. CREAMY DILL DRESSING MAKES CUP (125 ML)

This is also a good way to use up the fronds
from the end of fennel, and is lovely with fish.

½ cup (125 ml) Whey-Good Mayo
2 tablespoons dill or fennel fronds, snipped finely

Combine both ingredients and stir.

5. CREAMY GREEN DETOX SAUCE MAKES CUPS (350 ML)

½ bunch of watercress or 1 small bunch of coriander
juice of ½ lemon
½ cup (125 ml) Whey-Good Mayo

Purée the watercress or coriander in a blender or food
processor. Add the lemon juice and stir in the mayo.

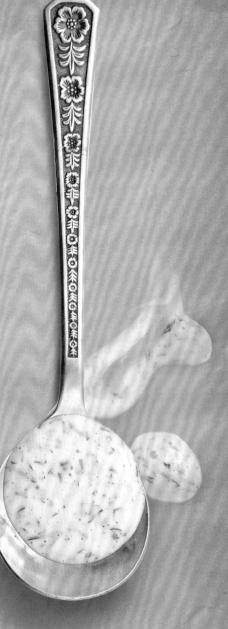
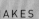

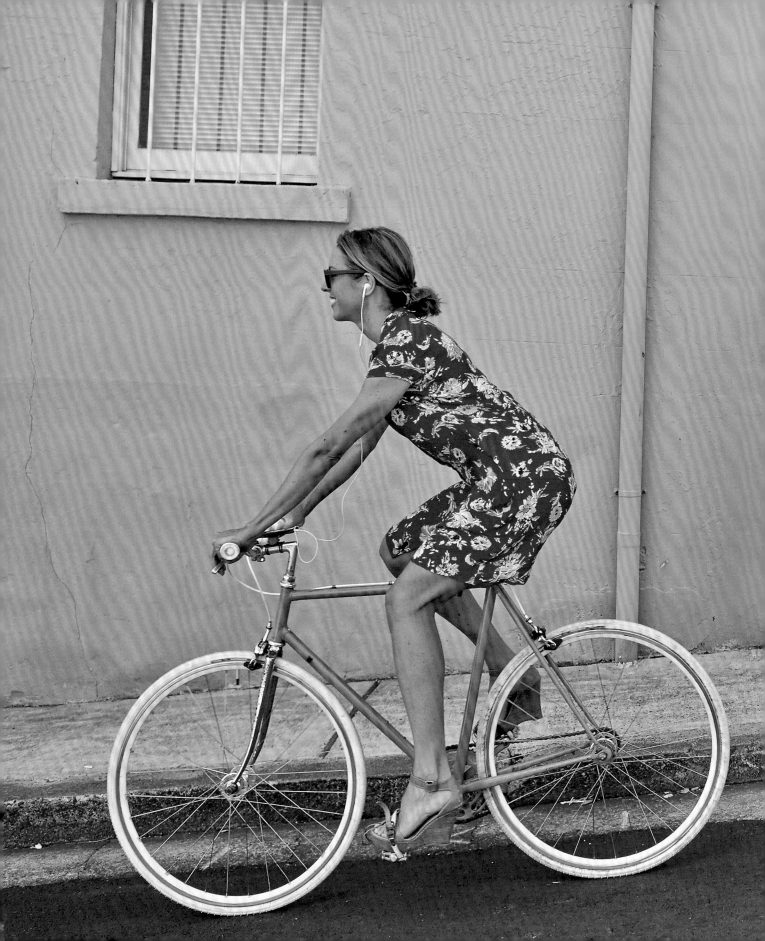

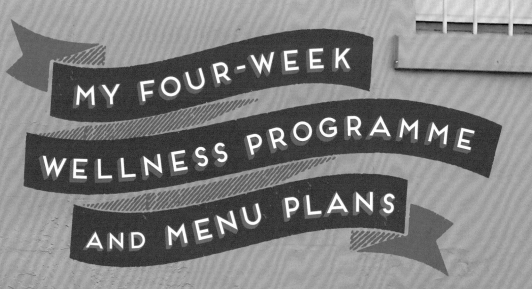

MY FOUR-WEEK WELLNESS PROGRAMME AND MENU PLANS

I've put together this snappy month-long reboot
and a bunch of different plans for those
of you who'd like a guided health programme.

IF YOU'VE PREVIOUSLY QUIT SUGAR BUT SLIPPED A LITTLE, OR IF YOU JUST WANT A HEALTH REBOOT, THIS PROGRAMME MIGHT JUST BE YOUR CUP OF ROOIBOS. I TURN TO IT WHEN I'M A BIT OFF-KILTER. It's designed to encourage you to find your own wellness flow, so that sugar-free living is sustainable, economical and low fuss.

But (and here I wave my arms wildly for emphasis!) it's not a strict programme; it's a series of experiments that allow you to get curious and playful so that you can establish what works for you. This is the whole point, yeah?

WEEK ONE

This week is about setting yourself up.

1. HAVE A BIG SUNDAY COOK-UP and fill your freezer with at least three of the below. This will entail going to a food market (check out primalbritain.co.uk/paleo-directory, or local-farmers-markets.co.uk). Buy produce that's in season and/or on special (and therefore abundant and cheap):

Feel free to tick off as you go

- ☐ Pumpkin Purée (see page 51)
- ☑ Sweet Potato Purée (see Pumpkin Purée variation on page 51)
- ☐ Par-Cooked 'n' Frozen Veggies (see page 51)
- ☐ Berries
- ☐ Fresh herbs 'preserved' in wine, oil or stock (see page 194)
- ☐ Green Glowin' Skin Smoothie ice cubes (see pages 76–7)
- ☐ Bone Broth – you might have to visit your local butcher in advance and ask them to set aside 2–3 kg of bones for you, ready for Sunday (see page 190)
- ☐ Activated nuts (these will take a few days, including soaking) (see page 204)
- ☐ Hamburger patties (Is mince on special? Discounted due to the Best Before date approaching? Stock up!)

2. COOK USING THE INDEX. Once you've got these staples in your freezer, flick to the Index and plan a bunch of meals to cook around these staples.

3. SHOP SMART.

- ☐ Find an online meat supplier in your area and bulk buy, filling your freezer with supplies for any of the recipes in the midweek One-Pot Meals (see page 109) and Reinvented Comfort Classics (see page 87) chapters.

- ☐ Research online speciality food providers (look for ones that deliver nationwide for a flat fee) and organic fruit and vegetable box delivery services (most major cities have these; Google 'organic fruit and vegetable deliveries' in your area). These are a great way to get stocked up on ingredients that are in season, local and (comparative to many other sources) cheap. Get started with these great links: riverford.co.uk, organicdeliverycompany.co.uk.

- ☐ Screen grab or print/write out the Shop Differently code (pages 42–4) and keep it on your smartphone or in your wallet.

4. CREATE A PERSONAL MORNING ROUTINE. Do the exercise on page 34. Play around with different approaches this week. What works? How long can you realistically dedicate to a daily routine? Write it down. Stick it to the back of your bedroom door or the fridge (eg: 'Every morning I spend 35 minutes starting my day right.') – and start this week. Every morning. Because it's the every day bit that counts.

5. DO SOMETHING DIFFERENT: TRY ONE OF THE SLOW-COOKED RECIPES. If you don't have a slow cooker, think about investing in one (they're super-cheap and available at most discount outlets; grab one in your lunch break) or you can follow the instructions on page 47 to use a standard pot.

☐ Slow-cooked Pork Belly Baked Beans (see page 64)

☐ Lemon and Cinnamon Lamb Shanks with Gremolata (see page 119)

☐ Slow-Cooked Barbecue Pork (see page 103)

6. INGREDIENT TO BUY AND TRY: Apple cider vinegar (from health food shops and most supermarkets). Have a tablespoon in hot water when you wake and, if you have any kind of digestion issues, before other meals during the day. Monitor how it affects your digestion and appetite. Does it make a difference? If not, use the rest of the bottle in the place of other salad vinegars, in the Slow-cooked Barbecue Pork recipe (see page 103) and other recipes in this book.

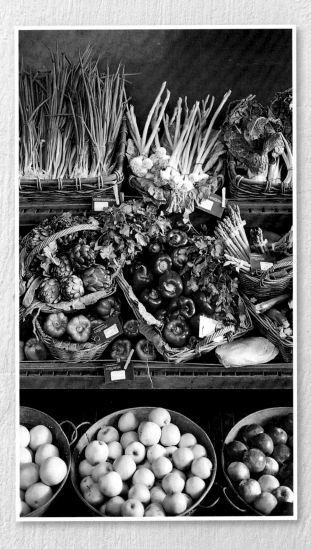

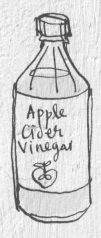

Apple Cider Vinegar

WEEK TWO

This week let's get any niggling cravings dealt with.

1. EXERCISE EVERY DAY THIS WEEK. Try at least 4 of the suggestions on pages 36–7 to make this happen. It need only be 20 minutes of walking, but for this week do it *every* day.

2. SWITCH AT LEAST THREE CAR OR PUBLIC TRANSPORT TRIPS TO A WALK.
The school pick-up or the dash to the corner shop for example. Did it work for you? Do the same trip again next week if so. Once a regular trip is easily done as a walk, it can become a habit.

☐ Trip 1

☐ Trip 2

☐ Trip 3

3. EAT AN EXTRA TWO SERVES OF GREENS A DAY.

☐ Try these side dishes, see pages 128–9 (two serves)

☐ Sneak some greens into a meal (one serve)

☐ Have a Green Glowin' Skin Smoothie on page 76 (two serves)

4. TRY SOMETHING DIFFERENT. Eat breakfast in a jar. This week prepare at least three of the breakfasts in the Totally Tote-able chapter (see page 71). Establish which works for you. Make two servings at a time and consume on consecutive days.

5. INGREDIENT TO TRY. A new kind of oil that you haven't tried before. Visit a health food shop to find macadamia oil and coconut oil for adding to your vegetables. At the supermarket or deli, try an infused olive oil – truffle, garlic, chilli – or look out for other interesting safe oils, like avocado oil.

WEEK THREE

This week is about upping the ante on flow and resourcefulness.

1. STOCKTAKE YOUR FRIDGE. Clean out everything – yes everything – and repurpose it (see the Brilliant Leftovers chapter on page 187 for ideas on how to use your leftovers), freeze it (see page 48–9), make a green smoothie or a mish-mash meal. While you're at it . . .

2. MAKE A FRIDGE SURPRISE. Your mission – should you choose to accept it – is to not have to buy any new ingredient for this one meal (see page 48). Hint: My Grounding Roots Winter Soup (see page 114) provides a good template for making a mish-mash leftovers soup.

3. EAT THREE MEALS A DAY ONLY (STOP SNACKING). To do this successfully and not go crazy with hankerings mid-meal, try all of the below this week (one at a time to see what works best for you):

☐ Buy a jar of organic, cold-pressed coconut oil and eat 1 tablespoon at the end of the meal, see page 16.

☐ Focus on having a bit of extra fat with every meal. Add a tablespoon of butter or oil to your vegetables or salad.

☐ Eat your (sugar-free, nutrient-dense) snack *with* your meal.

4. TRY SOMETHING DIFFERENT. An eating experiment. Give one of the following techniques a crack to see if it suits your eating style (try it for two weeks, then try another if it doesn't suit and you're still curious). But be sure to read up on the science behind each approach first, and heed any health advice I or other sources suggest. Also, be honest with yourself. If it doesn't feel right, abort and move on. I suggest doing them in this order:

☐ A 14–16 hour fast (see page 21)

☐ Limiting gluten (see page 22)

☐ Limiting carbs (see page 23)

5. INGREDIENT TO TRY. A 'daggy' or unfashionable food item. Perhaps one of the following (you can turn to the Index to find a recipe):

☐ Sardines

☐ Swede, chicory, kale, daikon, Brussels sprouts

☐ Secondary cut of meat (shanks, chicken thighs)

WEEK FOUR

Just some more experimenting that takes things to the next level . . .

1. DO A BULK-COOKING SERIES starting with one of the following (adding your own twists to extend things on and on). Start on a Sunday afternoon so you can get organised.

☐ A whole organic chicken (I've outlined how I do it on the next page). Use this as a template to do something similar with the options below.

☐ Lemon and Cinnamon Lamb Shanks (see page 119), which can be made into Lamb Shank One Pot Pasta (see page 120), Shanky Shepherd's Pie (see page 121) and perhaps a leftover lunch.

☐ Full-fat organic plain yoghurt to make cream cheese and whey; perhaps building to make your own mayonnaise or sauerkraut, or Gingerade (see the Ferments chapter, page 197) and the Yule Mule Cocktail (see page 146).

2. MAKE A DRESSING AND EXTEND IT. Try one of the following:

☐ Make Dressing in a Jar (see page 205) and extend it to make two extra flavours, storing each one in separate jars that you can roll out over your Great Grated Salads (see pages 82–3)

☐ Make the Whey-Good Mayo (see page 208) and extend it to make two extra flavours (you'll need to have made the cream cheese and whey to do so).

What now? Repeat from the beginning if you like, experimenting further, instilling deeper habits.
I wish you well . . .

3. TRY SOMETHING DIFFERENT. Get calm and balanced. I truly believe flowing, dense wellness for life is about getting balanced and happy with yourself and how you're conducting your own orchestra. Quitting sugar is a really good first step as it gets you clean and clear. But keeping things on track requires little refinements. Can I suggest you try any (preferably all) of the below as you get time:

☐ An infrared sauna

☐ Meditating (check at sarahwilson.com for tips)

☐ No stimulants (coffee, tea, cacao, cocoa)

☐ Going to bed by 10 pm

☐ Cooking gently. Use the cooking process as a time to get mindful. Heat your food low and slow.

INGREDIENT TO TRY. Sauerkraut. This stuff is the bomb. You can make your own, of course, see page 200. Or you can buy in speciality and health stores. However: ensure it's fermented in brine or whey (the ingredients should only be vegetables and salt and/or whey) and not pickled with vinegar and sugar. See if it enhances your meal and gut happiness.

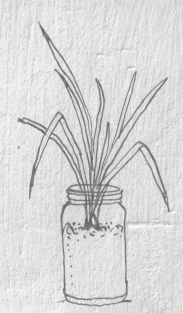

ONE CHOOK, FIFTEEN MEALS

OH, THE FUN YOU CAN HAVE WITH THIS CHOOSE-YOUR-OWN-ADVENTURE CHALLENGE!

To play, it entails starting with one (bulk-cooking) dish, then dragging out the various leftovers, scraps and by-products from there.

An organic chicken ain't always cheap. But you can make it work for you by extending it to create a number of different meals.

2 I then take the leftovers to make the **ROAST DINNER GRATIN** (see page 113) for the next day. Makes: 1 serve.

1 For instance, I start with a whole chook and make **CRISPY ROAST CHOOK** (see page 111). Makes: 4 serves.

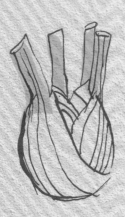

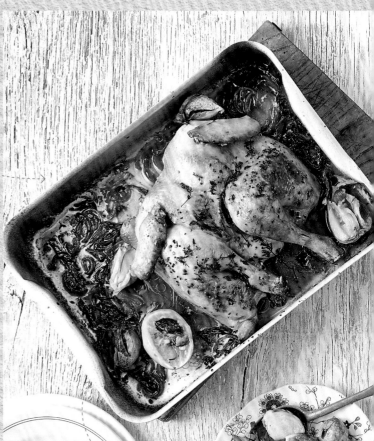

3 And any leftovers, which I keep in an ice-cube tray, are used to cook my next **CRISPY ROAST CHICKEN.**

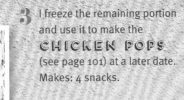

3 I freeze the remaining portion
and use it to make the
CHICKEN POPS
(see page 101) at a later date.
Makes: 4 snacks.

4 The carcass from the roast is then
used to make **LEFTOVERS
CHICKEN STOCK**
(see page 191). Makes: 1.5 litres (6 serves).

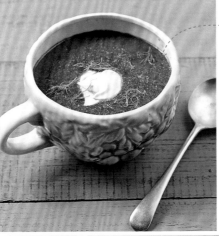

5 Some of the stock is used to make
**SWEET FENNEL AND
BEETROOT LEAF
SOUP** (see page 188) the
following week.

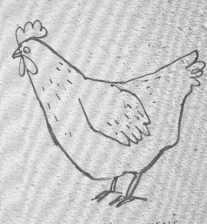

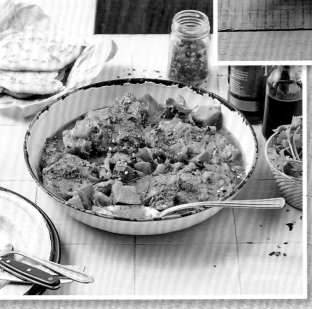

6 Some of the stock is used to
make **VIETNAMESE
CHICKEN CURRY**
(see page 122).

THAT'S 6 CONNECTED MEALS
— 15 SERVES —
FROM THE ONE CHOOK!

7 I'll then drink a cup of the
stock on its own, for an
energy kick.

MENU PLAN FOR FOURSOME FAMILIES

This eating plan is geared at families and groups of four (perhaps share houses). I've planned it so that some of the batch recipes can be done on a Sunday with the kids or housemates or . . . your dog, so that they can then eat them in lunchboxes the following week.

For lunch, add in the items from A Week of Lunchbox Ideas (see pages 166–7).

Some Other Good Things to Know:

► Make sure you double the smoothie and whip recipes to make 4.

► There are also five slow-cooker recipes. You can prepare the night before/that morning and let it cook while you're at work/school.

► For some low-fructose sugar options, check out iquitsugar.com.

► The weekend prior: you might like to . . .

☐ Make a batch of Deceptively Sweet Chilli Sauce. It can then be used on the 'One-Pot Wonder' Sweet Chilli Jam and Cashew Fish, Cauliflower 'Fried Rice' and Baked Satay Chicken Pops.

► On Sunday: you might like to spend the day making a bunch of fun things for the following week's lunchbox:

☐ Make double quantity of the Paleo Inside-Out Bread, slice and freeze in batches of two in zip-lock bags. The LCMs can also be used in lunchboxes.

☐ Make a batch of Raw Breakfast Balls.

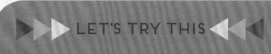

LET'S TRY THIS

OUR DIETITIAN SAYS:

'This plan exceeds the recommended dietary requirements for protein, vitamin A, riboflavin, niacin, vitamin C, phosphorus, zinc and omega-3 fatty acids providing families with an abundance of immune and brain boosting nutrients. These counts were calculated using the lunchbox suggestions from page 166–7.'

FAT: 47% PROTEIN: 25% CALORIES: 1300

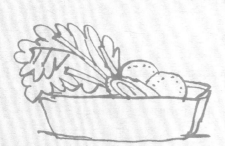

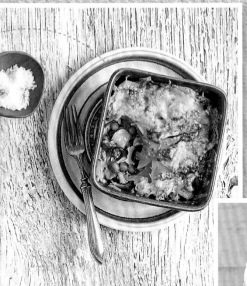

3 I freeze the remaining portion and use it to make the **CHICKEN POPS** (see page 101) at a later date. Makes: 4 snacks.

4 The carcass from the roast is then used to make **LEFTOVERS CHICKEN STOCK** (see page 191). Makes: 1.5 litres (6 serves).

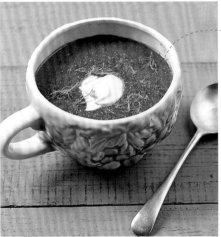

5 Some of the stock is used to make **SWEET FENNEL AND BEETROOT LEAF SOUP** (see page 188) the following week.

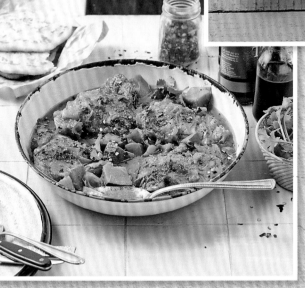

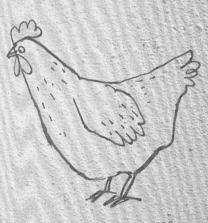

6 Some of the stock is used to make **VIETNAMESE CHICKEN CURRY** (see page 122).

THAT'S 6 CONNECTED MEALS — 15 SERVES — FROM THE ONE CHOOK!

7 I'll then drink a cup of the stock on its own, for an energy kick.

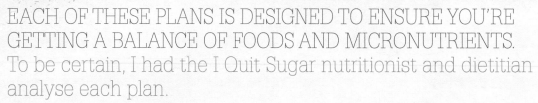

EACH OF THESE PLANS IS DESIGNED TO ENSURE YOU'RE GETTING A BALANCE OF FOODS AND MICRONUTRIENTS. To be certain, I had the I Quit Sugar nutritionist and dietitian analyse each plan.

You'll note the plans are low-calorie (the recommended daily intake is 2000 for women, 2500 for men). This is to allow you to add extra fat, to taste. I advise adding additional oils, cheese, nuts, avocado, etc. at most meals, according to your appetite needs, as you know by now.

MENU PLAN FOR BUSY SOLOS

This is a two-week plan because it entails cooking up in bulk and freezing things that can be eaten later in the fortnight (and beyond). Cos that's how we roll!

Some Other Good Things to Know:

► I plan salads and the use of fresh veg early in the week, soups and leftovers meals at the end (to use up fridge dregs).

► I've structured the plan so that batch items can be cooked at the weekend, ready for the week.

► The weekend prior you might like to:

☐ Buy prawns for two meals (3 serves).

☐ Grate the cauliflower in advance and freeze in 2-serve bags.

☐ Make a batch of activated nuts and seeds (see page 204).

► On Monday:

☐ Make Great Grated Salad to serve 4 and divide into jars, ready to add different dressings and additions.

► On Tuesday evening or Wednesday:

☐ Make chicken stock using the chicken carcass.

► On Thursday:

☐ You might like to make up the patties for the Deconstructed Hamburger, while making the Meatza, and freeze ready for the following week.

► There are also two slow-cooked recipes that you can prepare the night before/that morning and let cook while at work or school.

THE BEST GREENS FOR SOLO COOKERS
(so there's less wastage and fuss)

► broccolini (tenderstem broccoli) and asparagus (a bunch can go between two meals, or for dinner and lunch the next day)

► courgettes (one works tidily between two meals, along with a second veg)

► beans, mangetout, Brussels sprouts and prepared squash: buy by the serve.

► big things like broccoli and cauliflower: par-cook and freeze.

► a small bag of coleslaw mix (can stretch across 2–3 meals)

►►► LET'S TRY THIS ◄◄◄

OUR DIETITIAN SAYS:

'This menu is densely nutritious and vegetable-based, exceeding all micronutrient recommended daily intakes, including 2.5 times the RDI for riboflavin and niacin and 4.3 times the RDI for vitamin C, which provide antioxidant, anti-inflammatory and anti-ageing properties. It adheres to the optimal macronutrient ratio suggested by Paul Jaminet in *Perfect Health Diet*. This is considered the best default ratio by many health professionals.'

FAT: 51% PROTEIN: 26% CALORIES: 1400 (excluding snacks)

WEEK ONE

I like to tote hard-boiled eggs and eat with pepper and salt.

MONDAY	TUESDAY	WEDNESDAY	THURSDAY	FRIDAY	SATURDAY	SUNDAY
Sweet, Clean Protein Machine (page 77) plus 2 tablespoons activated nuts or nut butter (straight from the jar)	Sweet, Clean Protein Machine (page 77) plus 2 eggs, any style, on toast (optional)	Paleo Choc-Coco Muggin (page 66)	Carrot Cake Porridge Whip (page 72)	Carrot Cake Porridge Whip (page 72)	2 eggs, any style, with toast (optional), avocado, spinach, feta (at home or out)	Berry Omelette (page 68)
Prawn Cocktail Mish-Mash Great Grated Salad (page 83)	Rainbow Great Grated Salad (page 83)	Vietnamese Chicken Great Grated Salad (page 83)	Leftover Cauliflower 'Fried Rice' (page 100)	Middle Eastern Meatza (page 97), with 2 serves greens	Strawberry and Avocado Toastie (page 56)	2 Mexican Nacho Meffins (page 58) (with avocado icing or simply serve with half an avocado, sliced, and cherry tomatoes, halved)
Thai Red Curry 'Bolognaise' with Thai–talian Salad (page 106)	Crispy Roast Chook with Sweet Potato Casserole (page 111)	Cauliflower 'Fried Rice' (page 100)	Middle Eastern Meatza (page 97), with 2 serves greens	Grounding Roots Winter Soup (page 114)	Lemon and Cinnamon Lamb Shanks with Gremolata (page 119), with Cauliflower Cream (page 100) or puréed sweet potato, and 1 serve greens	Roast Dinner Gratin (page 113) with 2 serves greens

Make 4 serves of the meat sauce, freeze 3 portions.

Remember to make stock after dinner!

WEEK TWO

MONDAY	TUESDAY	WEDNESDAY	THURSDAY	FRIDAY	SATURDAY	SUNDAY
I am Graceful (Anti-Inflammatory Blend) Smoothie (page 77) plus 2 tablespoons activated nuts or nut butter (straight from the jar)	I am Graceful (Anti-Inflammatory Blend) Smoothie (page 77) plus 2 eggs, any style, on toast (optional)	Up 'n' Go Breakfast Whip (page 84)	Up 'n' Go Breakfast Whip (page 84)	2 Mexican Nacho Meffins (page 58)	Strawberry and Avocado Toastie (page 56)	2 eggs, any style, with toast (optional), avocado, spinach, feta (at home or out)
Roast Dinner Gratin (page 113) with 2 serves greens	Deconstructed Hamburger (page 88)	2 Mexican Nacho Meffins (page 58) plus avocado, cucumber and cherry tomatoes	Lamb Shank One-Pot Pasta (page 120)	Grounding Roots Winter Soup (page 114)	CHOOSE YOUR OWN ADVENTURE HERE: COOK UP SOMETHING YOU'VE GOT IN YOUR FREEZER	Pumpkin Pikelets (page 191) with yoghurt and toppings
Deconstructed Hamburger (page 88)	'One-Pot Wonder' Sweet Chilli Jam and Cashew Fish (page 124)	Lamb Shank One-Pot Pasta (page 120)	My Anti-Anxiety Soup (page 112)	Thai Red Curry 'Bolognaise' with Thai–talian Salad (page 106)	One-Pan Sardines 'n' Roots (page 116), with 2 sides greens PLUS Thyme 'Honey' Haloumi for dessert (page 159)	Slow-Cooked Barbecue Pork (page 103), with Cauliflower Cream (page 100), and 2 serves greens

NOTE: At the end of this fortnight you will have extra portions of chicken stock, Grounding Roots Winter Soup and Thai Red Curry 'Bolognaise' sauce, Meatza bases, pulled pork and hamburger patties.

NOTE: Make 2 serves (double the recipe)

MENU PLAN FOR FOURSOME FAMILIES

This eating plan is geared at families and groups of four (perhaps share houses). I've planned it so that some of the batch recipes can be done on a Sunday with the kids or housemates or . . . your dog, so that they can then eat them in lunchboxes the following week.

For lunch, add in the items from A Week of Lunchbox Ideas (see pages 166–7).

Some Other Good Things to Know:

▶ Make sure you double the smoothie and whip recipes to make 4.

▶ There are also five slow-cooker recipes. You can prepare the night before/that morning and let it cook while you're at work/school.

▶ For some low-fructose sugar options, check out iquitsugar.com.

▶ The weekend prior: you might like to . . .

☐ Make a batch of Deceptively Sweet Chilli Sauce. It can then be used on the 'One-Pot Wonder' Sweet Chilli Jam and Cashew Fish, Cauliflower 'Fried Rice' and Baked Satay Chicken Pops.

▶ On Sunday: you might like to spend the day making a bunch of fun things for the following week's lunchbox:

☐ Make double quantity of the Paleo Inside-Out Bread, slice and freeze in batches of two in zip-lock bags. The LCMs can also be used in lunchboxes.

☐ Make a batch of Raw Breakfast Balls.

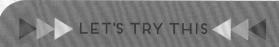
LET'S TRY THIS

OUR DIETITIAN SAYS:

'This plan exceeds the recommended dietary requirements for protein, vitamin A, riboflavin, niacin, vitamin C, phosphorus, zinc and omega-3 fatty acids providing families with an abundance of immune and brain boosting nutrients. These counts were calculated using the lunchbox suggestions from page 166–7.'

FAT: 47% PROTEIN: 25% CALORIES: 1300

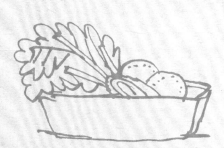

WEEK ONE

Make enough for 2 days' worth

Make double the amount and pour into drink bricks and freeze for lunchboxes during the week.

MONDAY	TUESDAY	WEDNESDAY	THURSDAY	FRIDAY	SATURDAY	SUNDAY
Up 'n' Go Breakfast Whip (page 84)	Low-fructose cereal with Green Glowin' Skin Smoothie (pages 76–7)	Low-fructose cereal with Green Glowin' Skin Smoothie (pages 76–7)	Up 'n' Go Breakfast Whip (page 84)	Snickery Pumpkin Mud Smoothie (page 74)	Strawberry and Avocado Toastie (page 56)	LCM Bars (page 152) with Green Glowin' Skin Smoothie (pages 76–7)
					Fennel Tarte Tatin (page 127)	Paleo Inside-Out Bread (page 61)
'One-Pot Wonder' Sweet Chilli Jam and Cashew Fish (page 124)	Lemon and Cinnamon Lamb Shanks with Gremolata (page 119), with Cauliflower Cream (page 100), and 2 serves greens	Cauliflower 'Fried Rice' (page 100)	KFC (page 92)	Lamb Shank One-Pot Pasta (page 120), with 2 sides of greens or salad	Slow-Cooked Pork Belly Baked Beans (page 64) PLUS Mango Weis-ish Bar for dessert (page 154)	Crispy Roast Chook with Sweet Potato Casserole (page 111) plus 2 serves greens

Double the recipe and serve drumsticks in lunchboxes tomorrow.

You might like to double the recipe and freeze half to eat next week.

Remember to make stock after dinner!

WEEK TWO

MONDAY	TUESDAY	WEDNESDAY	THURSDAY	FRIDAY	SATURDAY	SUNDAY
2 Raw Breakfast Balls (page 68) with 1 sliced kiwifruit or ½ cup (75 g) berries	2 Raw Breakfast Balls (page 68) with 1 sliced kiwifruit or ½ cup (75 g) berries	Low-fructose cereal with Green Glowin' Skin Smoothie (pages 76–7)	Low-fructose cereal with Green Glowin' Skin Smoothie (pages 76–7)	Up 'n' Go Breakfast Whip (page 84)	Berry Omelette (page 68)	2 Flower Power Eggs (page 169)
					Slow-Cooked Pork Belly Baked Beans (page 64)	Grounding Roots Winter Soup (page 114)
Baked Satay Chicken Pops (page 101) plus 2 to 3 serves greens	Slow-Cooked Barbecue Pork (page 103), with Cauliflower Cream (page 100) and 2 serves greens	Vietnamese Chicken Curry (page 122) with 1 side greens	Middle Eastern Meatza (page 97) with 2 to 3 serves greens	Sustainable Fish 'n' Chips (page 90), with Slaw (page 92)	Grounding Roots Winter Soup (page 114) with toast (optional) PLUS Christmas Pavlova Trifle (page 144) for dessert	Korean Pork Tacos with Cucumber Salad (page 104)

You can serve with some Deceptively Sweet Chilli Sauce and a bunch of veggie sticks to add to the 'lollipop' vibe.

Make extra meringues to keep for afternoon tea next week (with berries).

MENU PLAN FOR CLEAN WEEK

Try this eating plan when you feel you need to really recalibrate.

It's all about getting in extra dense nutrition (green vegetables at every meal), foods that are good for healing the gut and foods that go easy on the digestion (no nuts or grains; plenty of smooth purées and soups).

You can choose to do just three days instead of the five. Over to you . . .

SOME ADVICE FROM ME:

► This is a low-calorie plan. Make bigger portions of each meal by adding extra vegetables and clean oils and protein to ensure you're eating enough. Don't be too afraid of quantities, so long as it's simple, clean food.

► Also, make sure you have a tablespoon of apple cider vinegar in some warm water or a fermented food with lunch and dinner.

► Opt for Whey-Good Mayo-based dressings on the salads, for extra gut-friendly love.

► Also see 'How do you Deal with Lapses?' tips on page 25.

► The weekend prior you might like to:

☐ Make a Crispy Roast Chook (see page 111) and freeze in individual portions and make Leftovers Chicken Stock from the carcass (see page 191). Or use a whole chicken and make stock from scratch, again, reserving the chicken (see my recipe on sarahwilson.com). If you're stuck, simply buy ¼ roast chicken (preferably organic) and commercial organic chicken stock from the supermarket.

☐ Make some Homemade Cream Cheese a good four days in advance of the week (to allow enough time to make the whey and the subsequent ferments, below). We'll avoid dairy this week, but this fermented product is something of an exception.

☐ With the leftover whey, make some fermented vegetables, such as Homemade Sauerkraut (see page 200), to add to at least one meal each day, or add to The Succulent Berry Gut Cleanser (page 77).

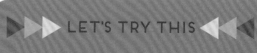

►►► LET'S TRY THIS ◄◄◄

OUR DIETITIAN SAYS:

'This menu is extremely balanced, in spite of being a "detox" plan, far exceeding all micronutrient recommended daily intakes, including 180% of the RDI for vitamin A and riboflavin, 550% of the RDI for vitamin C and 280% for omega-3 fatty acids, and is off the scale for gut-friendly probiotic bacteria. As Sarah urges, be sure to have extra large portions of the meals or some "clean snacks" on this plan to bring the calorie count to 1800-2000 if you're hungry or don't want to lose weight. Try a tablespoon of coconut oil (120 calories), ½ an avocado (150 calories), a handful of nuts (160 calories) or a green smoothie (150 calories).'

FAT: 45% PROTEIN: 32% CALORIES: 1100

Add a tablespoon protein powder
or leftover whey (per serve) and/or ½
teaspoon chia seeds for extra goodness.

DAY 1	DAY 2	DAY 3	DAY 4	DAY 5
I am Graceful (Anti-Inflammatory Blend) Smoothie (page 77), with 3 tablespoons Homemade Cream Cheese (page 204) with a sprinkle of cinnamon	I am Graceful (Anti-Inflammatory Blend) Smoothie (page 77) with 2 Flower Power Eggs (page 169)	The Succulent (Berry Gut Cleanser) Smoothie (page 77)	The Succulent (Berry Gut Cleanser) Smoothie (page 77)	Sweet, Clean Protein Machine (page 77) with 3 tablespoons Homemade Cream Cheese (page 204) with a sprinkle of cinnamon
Alkalising Great Grated Salad (page 83)	Vietnamese Chicken Great Grated Salad (page 83)	Not So Niçoise Cauliflower Pizza (page 98) with 2 sides of greens	Nourishing Kitcheri (page 63) with 1 side greens	Watercress Soup (page 85) with sardines and Homemade Cream Cheese (page 204) (simply mix 2 tablespoons of each, crumble and serve in chicory cups or on cucumber rounds)
Watercress Soup (hot or cold, page 85) with ½ cup (150 g) cooked prawns	Not So Niçoise Cauliflower Pizza (page 98) with 2 sides of greens	Nourishing Kitcheri (page 63) with 1 side greens	One-Pan Sardines 'n' Roots (page 116) with 2 sides greens	Grounding Roots Winter Soup (page 114) PLUS Hot Turmeric Milkshake (page 75) for dessert

You can make
two serves and
eat the second
one with lunch.

Take the soup
frozen to the
office to prevent
spillage.

Add plenty of fresh chopped
coriander and, for extra
Vata grounding, sweet
potato.

Note: make an extra serve
of sardines for tomorrow's
lunch.

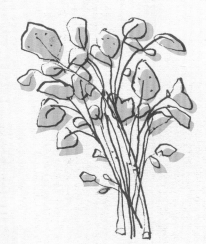

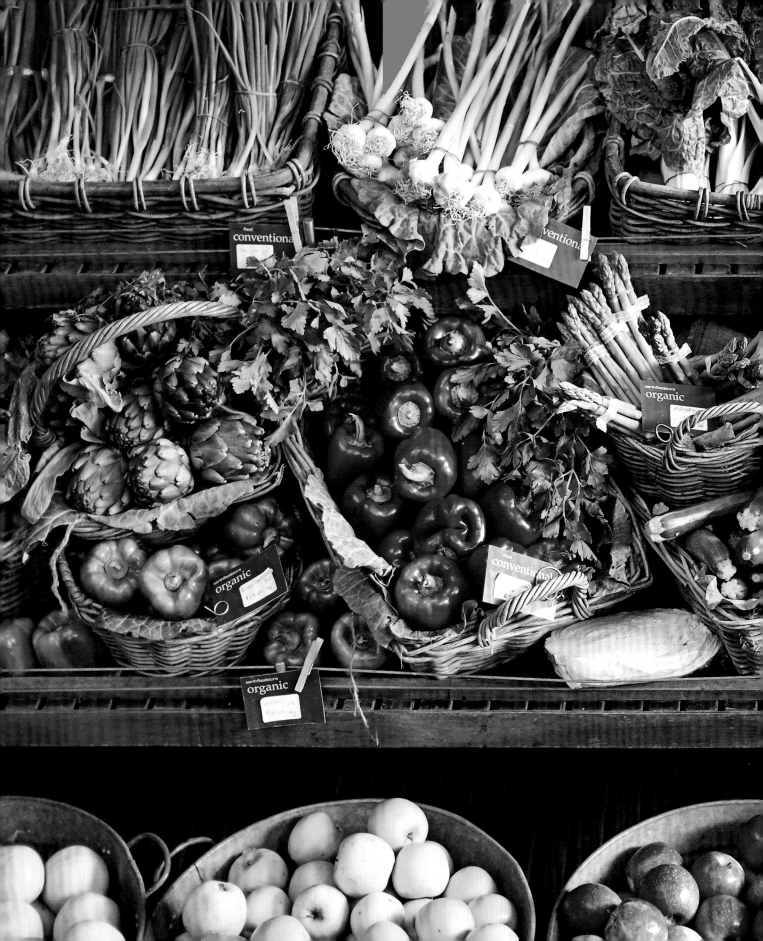

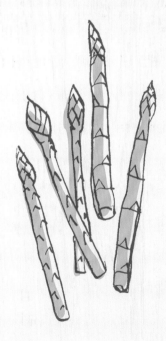

ABOUT THE AUTHOR

Sarah Wilson is an author, TV host, blogger and wellness coach whose journalism career has spanned 20 years across television, radio, magazines, newspapers and online. She's the former editor of *Cosmopolitan* magazine and was the host of the first series of *MasterChef Australia*, the highest rating show in Australian TV history. She appears regularly as a commentator on a range of programmes including Channel 7's *Sunday Night*, *The Morning Show*, *Sunrise* and *Weekend Sunrise*, Ten Network's *Good News Week* and *The Project*, Nine's *60 Minutes* and *A Current Affair*.

Sarah is an adept social commentator, following a career that's spanned politics, health advocacy, restaurant reviewing, opinion writing and trend forecasting. She's also a qualified Health Coach with the Institute for Integrative Nutrition in New York. Sarah's 8-Week Programme has seen over 280,000 people quit sugar.

She's also authored the best-selling series of ebooks from iquitsugar.com, including *I Quit Sugar: an 8-week program*, *I Quit Sugar Cookbook*, *I Quit Sugar Chocolate Cookbook* and *I Quit Sugar Christmas Cookbook*.

Sarah blogs at sarahwilson.com. Sarah lives in Sydney, rides a bike everywhere and when asked what her hobbies are cites 'bush hiking' , planning her next meal and being fascinated by other people with real hobbies.

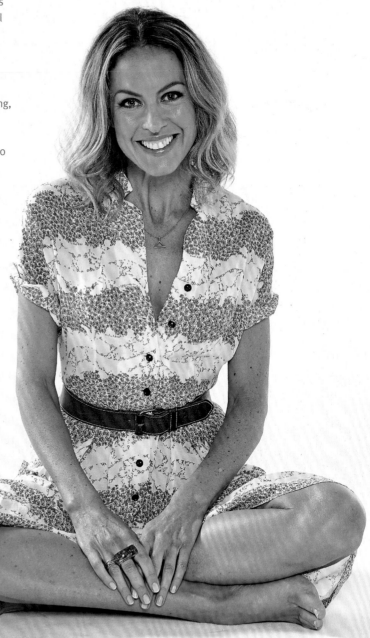

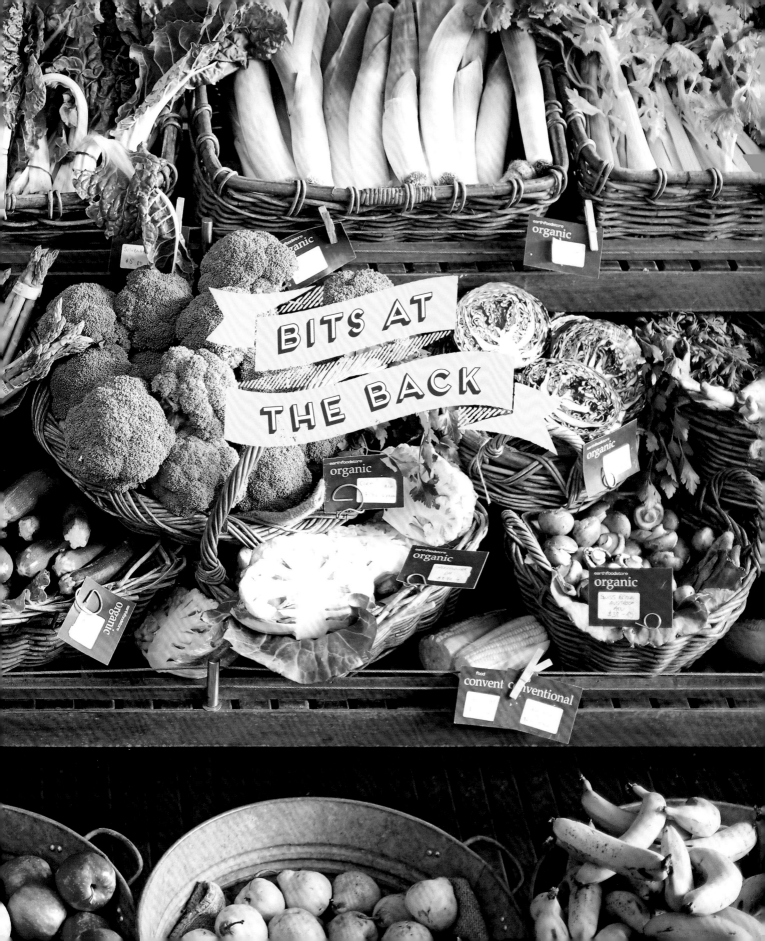

If you're wondering if it's good and right to eat meat ...

'Ordering the vegetarian meal? There's more animal blood on your hands', Professor Mike Archer, *The Conversation*, 16 December 2011, http://theconversation.com/ordering-the-vegetarian-meal-theres-more-animal-blood-on-your-hands-4659

Meat: A Benign Extravagance, Simon Fairlie, Chelsea Green Publishing, 2010.

The Vegetarian Myth: Food, Justice and Sustainability, Lierre Keith, PM Press, 2009.

'The China Study: fact or fallacy', by Denise Minger, Raw Food SOS blog, 7 July 2010, http://rawfoodsos.com/2010/07/07/the-china-study-fact-or-fallac/

'I was wrong about veganism. Let them eat meat – but farm it properly', George Monbiot, *The Guardian*, 7 September 2010, www.theguardian.com/commentisfree/2010/sep/06/meat-production-veganism-deforestation

If you're curious about whole foods, fermenting and slow cooking ...

Nourishing Traditions: The cookbook that challenged politically correct nutrition and the diet dictocrats, Sally Fallon, Newtrends Publishing, 1999.

Nourishing Traditions is my bible. It's dripping in all kinds of totally sound, 'just like my grandmother used to say' nutrition information about how we metabolise food. The high queen of the Weston A. Price movement, Sally really is the go-to on good gut health.

Cooked: A Natural History of Transformation, Michael Pollan, Penguin, 2013.

Cooked is a fun read on fermentation and slow cooking and a bunch of other foodie explorations. Follow him via the *New York Times* and @michaelpollan, too.

If you want to learn more about the latest science on sugar ...

Fat Chance: The bitter truth about sugar, Dr Robert Lustig, Fourth Estate, 2013.

Dr Robert Lustig, a paediatric endocrinologist, is your go-to on the latest science on sugar. His influential youtube video 'Sugar: the bitter truth' and seven-part series 'The skinny on obesity' is also worth a viewing.

Why we get fat: And what to do about it, Gary Taubes, Knopf, 2010 and *Good Calories, Bad Calories*, Gary Taubes, Knopf, 2007. Gary Taubes is an American science writer for the *New York Times*. He can also be found at garytaubes.com

Also go to www.iquitsugar.com/science where we outline the latest studies that draw on the highest standards of proof (meta-analysis and systemic reviews, randomised controlled trials and cohort studies).

And the whole 'which oil are we meant to eat' issue ...

Toxic Oil, David Gillespie, Penguin, 2013. David Gillespie is a pioneer of the fructose-free lifestyle in Australia who's moved his investigative zeal to the fat factor.

And for everything else ... you can follow me and the I Quit Sugar team as we curiously experiment at:

VISIT MY BLOG, **iquitsugar.com**
FOR ADVICE, TIPS AND TRICKS, RECIPES AND MORE.

FOLLOW ME ON TWITTER **@iquitsugar**

OR FIND ME ON FACEBOOK ON MY IQS PAGE
facebook.com/iquitsugar

CHECK OUT MY PINTEREST FEED FOR MORE RECIPE INSPIRATIONS
pinterest.com/iquitsugar/

I ALSO SHARE SUGAR-FREE FINDS ON INSTAGRAM

instagram.com/iquitsugar